Introduction

I'm no doctor, nor do I have any kind of degree related to the subject matter of this book. As such you are welcome to judge me accordingly but, a whole lot of people have changed the world and the way you live and they did not have degrees either. So I recommend you read this booklet first, before you judge me and I think you will see that a person does not need a degree to be smart, hard working, well informed, and indeed an expert in their field.

Although the horrendously overpriced rip-off colleges have not put me hundreds of thousands of dollars in debt, I am a consumer and I found myself looking down the massive vitamins and supplements aisle of a typical drug store and realized that there was absolutely no way a person could walk up, pick a multivitamin off the shelf, and get it right.

Furthermore, I realized that there was no way anyone could pick ANY product off of those shelves and get it right – that is, try to take something that would shore up what they perceive to be their weakness. And how could a person, like myself, even know what their weaknesses were in the first place?

This series of books intends to address this problem. I have done all of the research and I can tell you exactly which products have the best ingredients – which ones work – and where appropriate, which ones have such useless ingredients in them that they are worth avoiding.

And that's an important point, it is amazing to consider that some supplements on the very shelf I mentioned are almost completely useless, and it is amazing that they are even allowed to sell the garbage at all, but they are allowed to do it and we all know exactly why: greed and the insatiable thirst to steal that almighty dollar by the millions – the same greed, in the food industry that has made us all sick in the first place!

If we all stop buying the poisons that the greedy monsters want to shove down our throats, then they will stop wasting their time manufacturing those cancer cocktails and maybe they might actually start making products that are good for us.

One in three Americans will die of cancer, a disease that was one of the rarest known to medical science prior to World War II with only a handful – and I mean LESS THAN TEN – cases diagnosed by doctors each year. In the fifties these numbers exploded exponentially from hundreds per year to thousands to tens of thousands to hundreds of thousands of new cases each year. What changed? Two things: chemical additives to the foods we eat started appearing in the fifties and the nuclear bombs were set off in the mid-forties through the fifties. These bombs create what we all know very well as the mushroom cloud, this thing sends radioactive fallout as high as 30 miles, that's the edge of space, and the upper atmospheric winds can distribute that fallout world wide and it only takes ONE RADIOACTIVE ATOM to be absorbed by you, to ultimately possibly cause cancer in you.

We have no way of protecting ourselves from the radioactive fallout of those bombs or the Chernobyl and Fukushima disasters that have easily poured ten times the radioactive contamination into the Earth's atmosphere as all of the bombs before them did, but we can stop eating the POISONS that cause cancer and we can start eating the things that will make us healthier.

In the first two books the first chapter will be the same. The reason for this is that the information in it is so important that I have to include it in all of the books on the related subject matter of BEING and STAYING HEALTHY.

It would be incorrect if I were to say that clinical trials and studies are the ultimate evidence for proving something: they are not. And I would seem to be a hypocrite if I quoted you one study and said there's the proof and then scoffed at the next study. What I will do is this: I will quote you studies that indicate "No negative outcome." For example, if a study showed that feeding people a metric ton of some nutrient had no ill side effects, I will call that "conclusive evidence that the nutrient is safe." I will not quote a study that fed people a metric ton (far more than the normal and usual intake of a particular substance) and that then reported that the substance was toxic. The reason being that too much water is deadly (it is commonly known as drowning) so these reports are not necessarily of value to us. I will report a study that shows the efficacy of a substance. For example, if a bunch of people are dying of beriberi, and they are given a massive vitamin B complex and return to health, then it stands to good reason that the vitamin B complex worked.

On the other hand I will not quote a study that indicates that something is not effective. The reason for this again is that the study is not necessarily conclusive. For example, giving a massive treatment of a nutrient to people dying of cancer does not mean that the treatment has no usefulness if all of the people died because 1) We do not know what stage of the illness they were in (were they literally on their death beds already?) and 2) We do not know which particular cancer they had; there are roughly twelve major forms of cancer, you know a few of them like benign tumors versus malignant tumors, and tumors caused by a breakdown of the person's autoimmune system versus those caused by exposure to known cancer causing agents and so on. So some things might be highly effective against one kind and have no effect on another, but one thing is for certain: advising a person to stop consuming known toxins and to concentrate on eating healthy foods and taking vitamins and supplements, while it may not cure carcinomas, certainly won't do any harm either.

Three things are killing Americans:

1. They eat POISON in the form of CANCER CAUSING ADDITIVES to their PROCESSED foods on a DAILY BASIS. (And they are exposed to other POISONS also on a daily basis, like DIESEL ENGINE FUMES, HARSH CLEANER FUMES, etc.)

2. POOR DIET: even if you eat right, most of the plants are being grown in dead soil that has been overused for decades, the only reason the plants grow at all is because of the massive amounts of fertilizers being used on them – artificial, manufactured, chemical concoctions. This is what I affectionately call DIRTOPONICS. Just like HYDROPONICS or AEROPONICS, the plants must be given 100% of their nutritional requirements in order to grow, the only difference is that they are sitting in DEAD SOIL instead of pure water or air while they grow. Because of these conditions, many of the macro and micro-minerals are dramatically reduced or completely missing, having been absorbed completely out of the soil by crops decades ago. Even the current crops, manage to eek out an existence based on their fertilizer sources of nutrients but cannot possibly be producing the supplements we expect from them in the quantities that they should be producing, hence we are all malnourished even if we eat the right foods because they simply no longer contain adequate, or natural, levels of the nutrients that they should be providing us.

3. LACK OF EXERCISE: You cannot expect to be healthy if all you do is sit in your car on the way to work. Sit at a desk all day at work, and sit at your TV all evening when you get home. I'll talk about getting adequate EXERCISE in several volumes.

This series is designed to guide you through the bewildering maze of the essential nutrients and other supplements on the shelf at your favorite drug store and is not a substitute for professional advice. If you are currently on medication of any kind, you MUST CONSULT A DOCTOR before taking anything, including vitamins because they STRONGLY AFFECT the way your body works and could actually cause a VERY BAD REACTION in combination with certain strong medications.

Furthermore and of far greater importance, the series will show you how to eat properly, or rather, how to set up a regular food regimen that will provide you with all of the essential nutrients from natural whole foods rather than pills which have been shown in many studies to be far less effective than the whole foods they were extracted from or worse mimicked by pure synthetic replacements. More and more doctors and health professionalss are starting to recommend natural whole foods over purified extracts and manufactured chemicals, a realization that I have been advocating for thirty years.

Also, while I originally aimed this series primarily at vitamins and minerals, they are ONLY THE BEGINNING, there are a multitude of ESSENTIAL nutrients that are neither vitamins or minerals. These will be covered in an upcoming volume: The Truth About … MINERALS and ESSENTIAL NUTRIENTS.

Now, read and learn.

If you really want to be healthy, that is, if you are looking for the most effective vitamin/mineral/supplement, then you are interested in being healthy and staying healthy. And rule number one in working toward being healthy is to stop eating poison and to start eating foods that do not have a significant percentage of poison in their ingredients.

Now I cannot possibly list for you all of the poisons that the greedy moneygrubbers are putting into our foods – that would require far too much paper and make the book rather expensive, but I can give you a few examples and I think you'll get the idea and be able to identify poisons in your food with no trouble after that.

First a little chemistry, and I do mean a little. I'm no chemist, but I did study it in college and it was one of two possible choices for my major, the other was physics, but life and all of its problems, including health issues ultimately conspired to keep me from achieving my dreams. However, that was then, and this is now. And now that I have removed the greedy monsters from my life, a much healthier one now I might add, I can concentrate on bringing you the truth, not just about food, nutrients, and so on, but about everything.

Your stomach has one main function: to bathe everything that lands in it in a roughly pH 1 solution of Hydrochloric acid. This happens to be an incredibly dangerous and corrosive solution that while not as bad as alien blood (from the movie "Alien") it is one of the strongest acid solutions anywhere rivaling even the content of a car battery!

Anyway, the objective is to let that acid reduce complex molecules in the food into simpler ones and we're talking mainly about, fats, starches and proteins all of which get cut down into smaller chunks, so starches are turned into sugars, proteins into amino acids and so on.

What is interesting about our stomach solution is that many things can dissolve in it, and if they dissolve in the solution, then it is also likely that they can be absorbed easily, either through the stomach lining itself which while unlikely is possible, but definitely through the intestinal walls and with great ease if the substance has been dissolved in the liquid released by the stomach into the beginning of the intestines called the duodenum. This section of intestine is tougher than the rest and can reabsorb the Hydrochloric acid that is still in the liquid called chime (kyme) and get it out of there so it won't burn up the rest of your intestines.

Most, not all – we bear that in mind – Sodium salts will easily dissolve in the stomach acid. This frees the opposite piece in solution to be absorbed. For example, table salt is Sodium Chloride and it dissolves easily in the stomach solution yielding free Sodium ions and free Chloride ions. Both can be easily absorbed in the intestines thereafter. The Chloride ion is simply a Chlorine atom and you may have guessed from the nature of Hydrochloric acid, and the Mustard Gas used to kill thousands in World War 1 and the fact that adding it to your pool keeps microbes from infesting it, that this substance is TOXIC or in layman's terms: it is a deadly poison to almost all forms of life.

Trust me, the fish in the sea have fought for millions of years just trying to stay alive while swimming through it – it is a POISON. And you do not need this poison in your body. Therefore, do NOT eat too much salt. Sodium by the way is not good for you in excess either.

Now remember, just about anything that starts with the name Sodium, Sodium blahblahblahate for example, is SOLUBLE in your stomach. And granted, you actually do need some sodium in your body, what the sports drink people say they give you to replenish your "electrolytes," but you don't need tons of it and potassium and magnesium may be by far the better "electrolytes" over sodium anyway. Also remember that just about anything like blahblahblahium Chloride is also very likely going to be SOLUBLE = EASILY absorbed and also free up the POISON known as CHLORINE. Again, you need a little, so your stomach can actually manufacture the HydroCHLORIC acid it uses to continue your digestive process, but again, you don't need tons of this poison inside of you. Where does the excess of these things go anyway? Straight into the liver.

That's where every single molecule you eat goes by the way, through what the health professionals call affectionately, the HEPATIC PORTAL VEIN. Basically all of the capillaries in the walls of your intestines that are absorbing every molecule of what you ate gather back together into a big vein that feeds directly into your liver. This organ gets the first look at what you had for dinner, every time. This is how what you had for dinner gets regulated. Otherwise you would have dinner, say a steak and a potato, and the potato would be converted into sugars which would hit your bloodstream within half an hour and you'd be on the same sugar rush as if you had bolted down a two liter bottle of soda – that would not be a very good plan, and so that's why everything funnels into the liver.

The liver will grab up almost everything and then try to slowly release it back into the bloodstream over the next several hours, at least. And in the case of POISONS it does recognize an amazing number of them and tries to permanently take them out of circulation. You can bet it regulates the electrolytes since a particularly salty meal would likely cause you to have a heart attack if it didn't (the electrolytes are involved in the electrical field of the entire human body – the subject for a coming book, so you know – and dramatically affect the heart which does have a natural pacemaker by the way.) And you can bet it does everything it can, including letting its own cells DIE for the cause, in trying to remove POISONS from the blood stream coming from the intestines and you can bet that one of these is CHLORINE.

Now the liver can take some abuse along these lines and regenerate on its own, that is its job, but pushing it to its limits and beyond every single day leads to liver disease, liver failure, cirrhosis of the liver (too many cells have been killed repeatedly to the point where it can't grow back as fast as it is being destroyed by the POISON known as ETHANOL – usually – and so the liver literally dies a long slow horrible death and takes the overindulgent drunk idiot through a similar long slow and horrible death along with it.) Yes, you guessed correctly, ETHANOL, the alcohol in alcoholic beverages is one of the worst POISONS you can pickle your liver in – 4 to 6 ounces of alcohol (13% or less) in one sitting one time per day is acceptable for healthy individuals only. Any more than that and you are taxing your liver unnecessarily and that will come back to KILL YOU in the long run.

Ok, so what do we know? Sodium blahblahblahate and blahblahblahium Chloride are both likely very SOLUBLE in our digestive tracts but they will dump unwanted POISONS in the form of excess sodium ions, which the liver will try to regulate, but in the end will release into your blood and remember these are electrolytes and they can really mess up your electrical field and mess with your HEART which is why all the doctors scream, "No salt!" And the other extremely toxic one CHLORINE which is why they pump the tap water with a fraction of a percent of it which is good enough to kill just about every known microbe on Earth. Microbes are nothing more than single celled organisms … cells … cells that DIE when even a TRACE of CHLORINE is around. Oh yeah, you happen to be made out of cells … cells that die in the presence of chlorine – get it?

Now let's look at a few food label ingredient items shall we? I won't mention the actual food products I found these in, for fear of being mercilessly sued into dust by the greedy money worshipping owners of the companies that manufacture these beautifully packaged POISONS. Here are some of my favorite HORRORS that I have found in food – that you EAT:

1) SODIUM BENZOATE – This may be in every single packaged food product on Earth, or at least in the United States, as a "preservative." Well, it might keep the food the same color and texture for a longer period of time, but it is certainly not preserving the person who eats it. Case in point: Benzene, (the Benzoate ion simply has an oxygen atom bonded to it, which does help lessen its TOXICITY but it certainly does not make it into manna from heaven either) used to be found in every high school chemistry lab in the United States, including my own many years ago. But you won't find it there any more. Why? Because a lab did a study and

found that the vapors (it is highly volatile with a unique aroma, another such small organic molecule with a strange unique aroma is Napthalene or moth balls) and those fumes are extremely carcinogenic and we can't have the children being exposed to them can we? Absolutely not! But make sure they get their daily DOSE OF THE POISON in the meals they eat EVERY SINGLE DAY! Even if Sodium Benzoate's ion is 1/10,000th the carcinogen as the precursor Benzene, the fact is that every single man, woman and child in the United States eats this POISON almost on a DAILY BASIS. And the last time I checked 300 million divided by ten thousand is still 30,000; as in cases of CANCER. I don't want to be one of them, do you?

2) SODIUM CASEINATE – This is one of my favorites. Ever hear of Casein paint? Basically this food product had wall paint in it and the manufacturer had the audacity to put in parenthesis an explanation for why this ingredient was in the food: "added for texture." They added this garbage – house paint! – to give the food the right TEXTURE. Personally, I think I stopped wanting to eat paint by the time I reached the age of two years old, but thanks anyway.

3) SODIUM STEARATE – Another favorite, this is SOAP. Now I admit I've got quite the potty mouth, but my mother never washed my mouth out with soap, and as an adult I am not about to start either. These monsters didn't even have the decency to explain to me why they put the soap into my food either. Well I guess it keeps it clean right? Ever wonder why soap cleans so well? It bonds with fats and oils and is also soluble in water, this means that it grabs up the oils and dissolves with them into the water and then rinses away squeaky clean. Well I don't want all of my cells which are little bags of water and OIL to get rinsed away leaving my bones squeaky clean … I'd like to keep all of my cells right there where they are! This stuff is appearing on the rise in vitamin pills as Magnesium Stearate. It is almost impossible to find a pill that does NOT have it. Personally, I don't want to swallow a small chunk of soap, but it looks like they are giving us little choice in the matter.

4) YELLOW #5 – This is a particular pet peeve of mine. This well known carcinogen – and I mean there are plenty of studies explicitly showing this nuisance to be a verifiable cancer causing killer – is in almost as many things as that confounded menace Sodium Benzoate. This garbage causes cancer. Do not eat anything containing it and the manufacturers will eventually get the idea and stop using it.

5) The six major SUGAR SUBSTITUTES – acesulfame potassium, aspartame, neotame, sacharrin, sucralose, and sorbitol. I cannot speak for all of them but I can speak for some of them in particular. Saccharin is a well known cancer causing TOXIN, in fact it makes an excellent rat poison and roach killer. Personally, anything that

can kill a roach is nothing I want to be eating, these are the critters that survived the first thermonuclear bomb test. Aspartame has some studies linking it to cancer and so does sucralose. I think you're getting the idea: I'd rather risk rotting my teeth than dying of cancer. Now I know the diabetics are in trouble, they can't just go back to sugar. But that's ok, there are natural sugar substitutes and in their case they may have to consult with a doctor to see which ones will not mess with their blood sugar counts. As for the rest of us, do not bother consuming any artificial sweeteners, they cause cancer, period.

I understand that casein is a constituent of milk. Sodium caseinate is that ingredient likely reacted with sodium hydroxide (lye) to produce sodium caseinate. The problem is that any time a naturally occurring constituent in our food is CONVERTED from its NATURAL form into another compound, an ARTIFICIAL and UNNATURAL compound it is also converted from a USEFUL and HARMLESS constituent of our food into a USELESS and HARMFUL one.

Native Americans used willow bark tea for aches and pains. The pharmaceutical companies looked into it and discovered the "active ingredient" in that tea: aspirin. They learned how to synthesize it and produce pills of it and it works, but they have isolated a single constituent from the tea and sell it in a concentrated form. Aspirin is like listening to a single blaring trumpet while the tea is a complete orchestra playing a song. In other words, while the aspirin pill is the active ingredient and it does work, it also tends to punch holes in your stomach while willow bark tea does not. Even a natural ingredient isolated from the natural source and given in a pure concentrated form can transform the ingredient from a useful and harmless compound into a USELESS and HARMFUL one.

Now that you have several examples of additives to your food, what do they all have in common? They sound like they belong on the shelf of a college chemistry laboratory and NOT IN YOUR FOOD. And if it seems that way, if it sounds like that's the way it should be (those mad scientists experiments should be on the shelf of a lab somewhere, and not in your food) then chances are YOU'RE RIGHT. So read the label and if it contains anything I listed above, then it is automatically OUT, and if it has some other SODIUM blahblahblahATE or blahblahblahIUM blahATE in it – then DON'T EAT IT!

I guarantee you this: if the food product has an ingredients label, and is in a cardboard or plastic wrapped package then it has at least one of these manmade, manufactured CHEMICALS in it, and if man made it, it is thousands of times more likely to be POISONOUS, than if nature made it – even the same "exact" molecule and I'll tell you why right now.

No human being has ever SEEN an atom. There is evidence that they exist and I am not trying to deny that, what I am saying is that no one has ever gotten all the way down there to get a really good close up look at one. As such, there may be minute differences between one atom and another, in fact quantum theory confirms that, and there may be extremely subtle differences between two allegedly identical molecules, one made in a lab and the other made in a tree. There is scientific proof for this statement as well: sugar. You have heard of "left-handed" sugar before, right? It means that the molecule is large and extended in three dimensions like a shoe, it has length, width and height and a recognizable top side and bottom side and a characteristic, like the top view shape or bend in the shoe that makes the left one unique from the right one, and you can't just turn it over and use it, because your foot can't go through the bottom of the shoe in order to put it on, in other words, the left shoe and the right shoe are unique and cannot be interchanged, you will never want to buy a pair of shoes in which there were two left shoes in it, unless you actually have two left feet, of course. The same is true of the three dimensional shape of the sugar molecule and interestingly enough, all plants manufacture right handed sugar and they do not manufacture any left handed sugar. And in a laboratory, starting with say, carbon dioxide, and water (just like the plants do) humans could manufacture sugar, but without a differentiating enzyme (which I'll describe here) they would make 50% right handed sugar and 50% left handed sugar. The differentiating enzyme would be any substance used in the process of manufacturing the sugar that itself had only right handed molecules in it, that could then control the outcome and make all of the resultant molecules left or right handed. Whew.

One more statement concerning that: since we can't make exclusively right or left handed molecules from scratch (starting with molecules that do not have left or right handedness to them) then that differentiating enzyme would have to be collected from a living thing, because life has been doing this for eons. I'll mention "handedness" later on but suffice it to say that since WE are living things and therefore WE have a lot of exclusively left or right handed molecules in our construction and cellular processes, then it makes sense that at some point, if we encounter a quantity of the "wrong way" molecule, that it won't just be useless, but it might very well be POISONOUS to us as well. And there are such examples known to science, where the right handed one is good for us and the left handed one is bad for us.

Now I have had a rather lengthy excursion into this subject of left and right handed molecules and chemists call any molecule that has a sufficiently complex three dimensional shape that it can have left and right handed molecules "stereo-enantiomers" (YIKES! But now you've got yourself a nice $50 word to throw around at your friends!) And now I can return to my original point; there is no way for us to know all of the subtleties within molecules containing even five atoms, let alone dozens or hundreds and many molecules involved in nutrition are huge. Therefore, manmade, synthetic, artificial, whatever you want to call them, versions of molecules are not necessarily the SAME EXACT MOLECULES and can therefore be subtly different in such a way that they are SETTING YOU UP FOR DEATH, likely in the form of CANCER, and at the very least ARE HIGHLY INEFFECTIVE in the case of MANUFACTURED VITAMINS.

So what should you buy? Even if we cannot tell if the vitamins are from natural sources or if they have been manufactured, we can at least tell the difference between, USABLE FORMS and forms that are not so readily absorbed and used by the body.

Go to the produce section of your favorite grocery store and buy some fresh vegetables and fruits. Yes, they are all saturated in insecticides and fungicides and fertilizers and so on. But there is no stopping that unless you grow your own which I highly recommend by the way, or unless you pay plenty more to get "organic" produce. I'll discuss "organic" produce in an upcoming book too. Still, I'll side with the foods NOT BATHED IN SODIUM BENZOATE, SACCHARIN, and YELLOW #5 than those that are. Incidentally, I have found at least one food product that had ALL THREE of those in it. I am amazed that people don't fall to the floor, cold and hard, while partaking of that CANCER COCKTAIL.

What else can you eat? Go to the meats section and get yourself some chicken, or some fish. I grab a pack of pork chops when they are on sale (now and then, about once a month at most.) Contrary to popular belief, as long as you cook it well, it won't do any more harm to you in moderation than any other NATURAL thing made by the EARTH as opposed to those things manufactured by some greedy monster. It will certainly do far less harm to me than that little pink packet in your coffee.

Check the labels. Some brands might add things you don't want. If the chicken looks too yellow, guess what they have bathed it in? Yellow #5, you got it! Incidentally when I indict that garbage I am referring to ALL artificial food colorings and flavors, not just that specific one. Don't eat that POISON.

Yes, I know that most artificial flavorings are chemically "identical" to the real ones found in nature, but why is it that artificial grape flavored things taste nothing like natural grape flavored things? How identical are they? I believe I already warned you about this (sort of the same molecule not being exactly the same) and frankly I do not know how identical these molecules are to the natural ones, and I guarantee you that the greedy monsters POISONING YOUR FOOD with it don't know any more about it than the greatest physicists and chemists on Earth who would neither confirm nor deny my claims with anything more substantial than the Heisenberg Uncertainty principle, which supports my claim that they are different just as much as it would support their claim that undetectable differences are irrelevant. Sorry for the rant, but this stuff is KILLING US and if I get going down hill, there's no stopping me. The bad news is that the greedy monsters putting this manufactured POISONOUS CANCER CAUSING GARBAGE into our food DON'T CARE EITHER. "Just sit down, shut up, buy it and EAT it."

On rare occasion I buy canned goods and I do buy them for the purposes of having an emergency store of food, just in case the world ends tomorrow. I buy "No Salt" versions whenever possible and I buy one can and go home and open it. If the can is LINED, and not simply the raw metal, then I'll go back and get the twenty cans or whatever I intend to get. Even the canneries have figured out that when their food tastes like the can, people will go for the other product with the LINING in their cans so that their food does not taste like the can: and so most of them line the cans with an inert material like a thin plastic coating. It costs more to manufacture the cans with the lining than just making the cans without the lining so why do you think they bother doing it? Because WE THE CONSUMERS HAVE SPOKEN WITH OUR WALLETS on the subject and that is exactly what we can always do and make these monsters STOP POISONING OUR FOOD.

Back to the discussion, if the cans are lined then I buy the stuff. If the can is NOT lined, then very likely the contents do taste like the can, do not even give that stuff to the dog, throw it away and I'll tell you why.

It's called metal poisoning. You know, the thousands of dollars you have to spend for a licensed contractor to come in and strip your walls of lead based paint and repaint your house so you can actually sell it on the open market. Now, luckily the monsters that have elected themselves to be the ones to feed us all, have found cheaper metals than lead to put our food into or trust me they would do it. Still those metals are not necessarily better for you than lead either. And the one I am talking about in particular is aluminum. There are reports that aluminum poisoning may be related to Alzheimer's disease; another very rare illness that has now magically become a massive epidemic. Where did this thing come from? Aluminum cans, especially aluminum soda pop cans. This is the perfect storm: Aluminum in contact with a weak acid, Carbonic Acid, which in solution can form a strong base and suddenly grab up the aluminum molecules in the walls of the can and take them into solution as Aluminum Carbonate. Not necessarily tons of this; just a minuscule trace amount, but what if this garbage gets inside you and somehow gets trapped in your brain chemistry somewhere and NEVER GOES AWAY? Then tomorrow you suck down another pop, then another, and eventually, from accumulating the POISON over decades in your brain, you don't recognize yourself in the mirror any more. STAY AWAY FROM ANY HIGHLY ACIDIC substance in any UNLINED METAL CONTAINER. That would mean any fruit product in particular. Do I buy canned fruits? Yes I do, some of them come in unlined cans, and they hit the trash can and I make a note of the product so I will never buy it again in life.

I have a gallery of photos on my computer to remind me of what products have been designed to kill me so that I will never buy them again. I would love to share, but all those foaming mouthed billionaire monsters lurking out there would slowly lower their own mothers into the pits of hell just to make a nickel, and I am fairly confident they would do the same to me defending that nickel.

Now take a moment to consider the following: how long would you survive without air, in particular oxygen? A few minutes at most. We could therefore say correctly that gaseous oxygen is the ultimate and most essential of all nutrients. Without it a human body shuts down and dies within minutes. This is because the oxygen provides the "oxidizer" for our cells to burn fuel (sugars mostly) from which they derive the energy to function. No energy to function: no life, and the main organ that has by far the highest demand for oxygen is the brain and that's exactly why you die so fast without air, because your brain, properly functioning, is that which is conscious and is, in essence, you. It is fascinating to note that most of the rest of the body can get along quite well for extended periods of time without oxygen, but that is of no use when the brain, which is the person, dies so fast without it.

Now our respiration, our breathing which provides this most essential of all nutrients, only needs to take up oxygen (and get rid of built up carbon dioxide which is the result of the metabolic burning of the sugars in our cells) and nothing else; a very simple bodily function and requirement.

The point I am driving at here, is that although the process of eating is not as imperative as breathing, in that you will not starve to death in minutes if you stop (although some people eat as if they think they will) this does not change the fact that if you do stop eating, then you will die. Therefore eating is an imperative process, as imperative as breathing, even though the time delay between stopping it is much more protracted, the outcome is the same.

The major difference is that eating, which involves the consumption into the digestive tract of essential nutrients, is the opposite of the simplicity of breathing, in which we do it to take up one simple nutrient. In eating, we absorb gigantic collections of gigantic molecules in such profusions and complexities that we may never be able to fully analyze a complete and healthy natural diet consisting of fruits, vegetables, and animal products.

But although we may not be able to fully chemically analyze our nutritional needs, that does not mean that those needs do not exist and it does not mean that we should just throw our hands up and give up. All that this means is that the mad scientists will never be able to provide us with a George Jetson diet of nothing but completely artificially manufactured pills that will keep us healthy for a long lifespan.

What I ultimately want to convince you of, with this argument is that:

1. There can never be an adequate substitution for natural foods. You can certainly take a Vitamin A pill to make sure that you get enough each day, but carrots contain not only all the Vitamin A that you need, but they also contain beta-carotene which is a powerful anti-oxidant that helps defend your entire body and all of its cells from being damaged by free radicals or "oxidants." But this exact same substance can be easily converted by the body into more Vitamin A as needed: that's why I would recommend to anyone concerned about Vitamin A to eat carrots, as many as you like, you very likely will not overdose on beta-carotene although you certainly CAN overdose on pure Vitamin A.

2. By eating natural foods you will take in nutrients that no one even knows exist, but that the human body needs nevertheless. The more variety you have in your natural food diet, the more likely you are to take in something that your body actually desperately needs.

3. Cravings have been suspected for years to involve a method by which the body reports a serious deficiency to the brain, and the craving is the way in which the brain drives the person to get the missing nutrient. Listen to your cravings and more importantly, keep rotating and changing your diet from one day to the next so that you never fall short for more than five days in a row of anything your body might need.

4. We know that all of our food, especially in the developed countries, from the plants, fruits, vegetables, grains, to the livestock that feeds on these plants are seriously lacking in critical nutrients because of the long dead dirt in which they have been cultivated. But the grape still looks like a grape, so it has still been able to construct its cells in all of their amazing complexity despite these shortcomings and therefore it has constructed complex molecules, that the mad scientists still have yet to discover or understand, and that your body needs in order to survive and to thrive. So despite my warnings that the plants and animals we eat are deficient, that does not mean that they are devoid of nutritional value. You must eat as many all-natural items in as much variety as you can in order to maintain optimal health and you must avoid at all costs ALL fake food; manufactured and processed foods, because they are rife with

cancer causing poisons and the processing has destroyed most if not all of the potential nutrients in them as well.

END OF CHAPTER QUIZ

1. Which of the following is more likely to give you cancer (if you eat it):
   A.   Something that naturally grew out of the ground, a plant product.
   B.   Something that naturally grew up eating plants, an animal product.
   C.   Something that some greedy billionaire monster made his mad scientists whip up in a test tube that costs one cent less per ton to make, than it does to use a natural product in the food product.
   D.   All of the above

Answer: C. If you chose either A or B, then you have been hypnotized by the high tech world into hating nature. Nothing from the Earth will give you cancer. Yes, there are poisonous plants and dangerous animals, and that's why our ancestors all died finding that out so you and I won't have to die trying to make Poison Ivy tea or trying to ride a Bengal tiger. Get it?

2. Which of the following does NOT cause cancer?
   A. Saccharin
   B. Benzene
   C. Yellow #5
   D. Water

Answer: D. Water however is deadly in excess; it's called drowning. But seriously, all these chemicals and additives in the food are bad for you. The only reason they put Yellow #5, a known POISON, in your food is for the PROFIT because it is cheaper than using a natural product and the only effect it has on your food is the COLOR of it. Personally, I'd rather eat a white pickle than a DEADLY ONE. (Every pickle in every jar on every shelf in every store has that blasted cancer causing yellow #5 in it which has forced me to start making my own.)

3. Which is least likely to have a cancer causing agent in it?
   A. A bunch of cherries in the produce section
   B. A jar of maraschino cherries
   C. A jar of Cherry Jelly
   D. A package of Chocolate covered Cherries

Answer: A. Everything else has passed through the manufacturing plant and received its pretty packaging and labeling and along with that, its heavy dose of chemical DEATH additives.

CHAPTER 2 – THE PROBLEM WITH ALL DIETS

The main complaint I have always heard concerning diets is that they don't work or they take a little weight off and then the diet "hits a wall" and basically stops being effective far short of the person's target weight. Aside from the fact that Americans are the best fed and most MALNOURISHED population the world has ever seen, the actual problem with ALL DIETS is psychological.

Now I am well aware of the fact that some people really do have physiological factors contributing to their weight problem: mainly in the form of a genetic predisposition toward obesity, and that certainly is a challenge to overcome, but it CAN BE DONE. When I say that the problem with all diets is psychological what I mean is that a person has spent their whole life NOT on a diet and then makes the decision to lose weight and goes ON A DIET. So now they are ON A DIET and have specific expectations about it, and what's worse, they expect at some point to GO OFF OF THAT DIET and "get back to their normal routine." This mindset is exactly why ALL DIETS FAIL.

The second reason that all diets fail, is the habitual dependency on food which has been termed "comfort food" or "comfort eating." This is possibly the most significant problem in that it becomes a habit almost for the sake of something to do while sitting in front of the TV, for example. Either way, all of these issues must be addressed; you must FACE them head on before you can lose the weight.

I have a natural tendency to be obese. I got it from my grandfather on my father's side. When I get overweight I get a huge tire all the way around below my navel. I look like an upside down light bulb on two skinny bird legs. I look disgusting to be blunt about it. And that is important: I do look in the mirror and FACE REALITY. I am rather UGLY to begin with, and when I am overweight I look dreadful. Well, I am not going to spend a million dollars to have a quack chop on my face to try to turn myself into Brad Pitt (or whoever is the latest heartthrob – which also never works anyway) but I CAN TAKE THAT TIRE OFF OF MY BODY.

If you have ever gone on a diet, even if you are dieting right now, that is a VERY GOOD THING. You have made the right choice – to lose the weight – and you are making the effort to try to lose it. So you are both READY and WILLING to do what is necessary in order to lose that weight. So the only thing you are missing is to be ABLE to lose that weight.

In order to be able to lose the weight you need two things: 1) You must determine the CAUSE of your current physical condition: why are you overweight? And 2) HOW do you go about losing that weight? If you have already made the determination that you are unhappy with your weight and made the decision to fix the problem – you are both READY and WILLING, now you have to become

ABLE to lose it. And the first thing necessary for anyone to be able to fix anything is to determine the CAUSE of the problem. A mechanic can't fix your car until he figures out WHY it isn't working: he must determine the cause of the problem. A doctor can't heal you until he first makes a correct diagnosis as to the cause of your symptoms. And you can never lose the weight until you FACE the TRUTH about the CAUSE of your current condition: Where did the weight come from in the first place?

Americans right now in general live in despair, hopelessness, frustration and STRESS. Now, we all cope with this and everyone manages to find some way to live with these negative mental forces. The top two causes are financial and interpersonal relationship related. And the top cause of relationship problems is financial so really there is only one cause for all of this grief: MONEY. For some people the problem is a simple LACK of it, for others the trouble comes from a high stress job. They make a lot of money but it is not easy. Either way, one of the solutions to this stress that many people accidentally fall into is overeating. I am certainly not saying that this is everyone's problem and the root cause of YOUR particular situation. What I am saying is that you must devote some serious thought – soul-searching – to finding the CAUSE of your current situation. Once you FIND the cause, then and only then can you actually FIX the situation.

The important thing to remember is that no one is being judged here. Everyone has their own closet full of skeletons. And the very best way to deal with them is to face them with the intent to make repairs to one's life. Everyone OWNS their own mind so there is no reason to carry a closet full of dreadful skeletons around throughout life. These psychological troubles can be addressed and that closet can get cleaned out and the skeletons can be put in the ground where they belong.

In the mean time, the physical causes of obesity are simple: 1) Eating the wrong foods, 2) Eating too much, and 3) Inactivity. There is no way to deny the fact that everyone who is overweight is engaged in this lifestyle and has been for a long period of time. And this is the physical cause of the current situation. This is the physical manifestation of the psychological stress that has over time driven the person to eat the wrong foods in excess and most Americans do not engage in enough exercise to maintain good health either.

And a diet cannot fix the weight problem, because it cannot address the root physical causes of it. Sure it will direct you to eat better foods and to limit the amount of food you eat, but it doesn't address the lack of exercise, and because it is a sudden regimen imposed on the person for the purposes of losing weight – you GO ON A DIET – then it becomes an imposition and an interruption of your NORMAL lifestyle. And so you determine that you will SUFFER THROUGH IT until you achieve your target weight and then you will get off of that diet, let yourself out of that purgatory, and get back to your normal routine: and that was the cause of the problem in the first place. And suffering through the diet just to achieve the target weight is DOOMED TO FAILURE.

And even if it does work, the person then gets off of that diet and gains the weight right back again, and it comes back much faster than the time it takes to lose it. I know: been there and done that.

So the answer is simple: do not GO ON A DIET. Instead, CHANGE your NORMAL eating pattern from a very unhealthy one to a very healthy one. And you do not necessarily have to make this a sudden and dramatic change either. You can make this change gradual if you prefer. There is a good reason to make this change gradual. Any sudden and dramatic change to your physical sustenance can be a shock to your system and when that happens your body will fight back. And when it fights back concerning your eating pattern it manifests itself in the form of hunger and cravings and that leads to misery and it is completely unnecessary for anyone to suffer like that.

I used to eat at least one big bag – the "party size" – of potato chips and suck down a 2 liter bottle of cola while sitting in front of the TV every single evening. That alone was worth something like 3 to 5 THOUSAND calories of the most unhealthy terrible kind of food and drink possible. And that is why I ended up about 80 pounds overweight. I am a rather small framed short person so it looked terrible on me too. Putting a stop to that was NOT EASY I assure you. But I did it and you will have to take a hard look at your caloric intake and make the necessary adjustments as well.

The Food and Drug Administration (when I spell it out like that it certainly does sound FASCIST to me) has determined that the average American needs 2000 calories a day. But I am not the average American – no one is. I don't have 2.4 kids nor have 0.58 dogs either. This is just a ROUGH AVERAGE GUESS and has NOTHING TO DO WITH YOU. It is true that we burn most of the calories we eat just maintaining our rather high body temperature of 98.6° F. And it is true that some people have a much more active metabolism than others. And it is true that some people are simply big framed and have a tendency to be overweight. But you can still adjust your eating pattern to include healthier foods and the proper amounts of them and this will go a long way toward achieving your desired goal of losing the weight and BEING HEALTHY, not just for the few months you STRUGGLE to stay on a diet, but for the rest of your life.

I had a roommate who over a period of a year or two had gained a huge amount of weight. All he did was sit in front of the TV and suck down bags of chips and drink soda pop. He decided to put himself on a diet and restricted it to 500 calories a day. After a few weeks he brought it up that despite only eating 500 calories a day he was still gaining weight. So I told him that was not possible, he would burn those calories in a day just to maintain a body temperature of 98.6° F. He heartily agreed and so I asked him to describe this "500 calorie per day" diet. He said it consisted of two sandwiches a day; each one had one slice of salami, one slice of cheese, and two slices of white bread. And he would have a bag of store bought popcorn. I asked to see the bag. He brought it to me and it was JUMBO, it would probably hold two gallons of water. I read the label and it did indeed say 250 calories per serving I then did a little math and showed him that the entire bag held about 2000 to 3000 calories (8 to 12 of the so-called servings) so he was actually on a 3500 calorie per day diet. And I pointed out that on occasion he would wolf down a half gallon of chocolate ice cream which also claimed to be about 400 calories but which actually contained about 15 servings (that's 6 THOUSAND CALORIES IN ONE SITTING!) I also pointed out that sitting around and doing nothing all day was not helping his cause at all.

He cut the junk food back to smaller portions and only on the weekend. And he started riding his bicycle a few miles a day and he started walking our other roommate's dog twice a day. And miraculously, the weight came off.

The point is that he forgot to take into account the fact that the label wasn't indicating the total calories of the food in the entire package, just a "serving" which was purposely SMALL, much smaller than what the average person was going to eat from it in a single sitting. And calorie counting is not as effective as one would think anyway. Any person who has a weight problem has become accustomed to consuming FAR TOO MANY calories on a daily basis. And when they start a diet and suddenly start counting calories and trying to stay under 2000 per day they quickly realize that for them, it is a CRASH STARVATION DIET. And they spend all day every day HUNGRY. And it is a terrible and MISERABLE feeling.

So it is impossible to really determine how many calories YOUR body needs. People with hard long strenuous days of labor might need 3000 calories a day while others who spend all day stuck in a cubicle answering phone calls might only need 1800. The point is that rather than try to figure out how many calories you need and instantly adjust to a dramatically different and dramatically reduced amount of food per day – to GO ON A DIET – from one day to the next is both tortuous and unnecessary and very likely to fail in the long run.

Furthermore, this mythical 2000 calorie LIMIT does not say what FORM these 2000 calories should be in either. Should it be a 2000 calorie brick of pig lard? Or perhaps it should be 2000 calories of tooth rotting soda pop that does nothing but punch holes in your stomach? Or maybe I will go on a 2000 calorie per day diet of nothing but steak. The point is that food contains a lot of different substances and we cannot even classify it into simple terms like "protein" or "fat" or "carbohydrates." One of the most irritating words I hear all of the time is "carbohydrates." A doctor for example might advise someone to avoid carbohydrates.

Personally, I would like to know how to do that. All life on Earth, and EVERY MOLECULE in EVERY CELL of that life is made out of Carbon, Hydrogen and Oxygen with some Nitrogen thrown in there as well. Carbon, Hydrogen and Oxygen ARE the definition of the term CARBOHYDRATE. "Carbo" is the carbon of course and "-hydr-" is the hydrogen and the "-ate" ending means oxygen. Now if EVERY SINGLE MOLECULE out of which EVERY STRUCTURE IN EVERY CELL is a CARBOHYDRATE of some form, then how does one reduce the amount of carbohydrates one eats? I suppose you could eat saw dust – oh, but wait, that's CARBOHYDRATES TOO!

The only way to reduce carbohydrates is to not eat anything that was ever alive: no plant products and no animal products because FATS are carbohydrates in their purest form (almost no nitrogen in them) and proteins are carbohydrates but they do have much more nitrogen and other things like sulfur and phosphorus in them. So you would have to drink water and eat plastic. Many packaged and processed foods might actually be nothing more than plastic, but they are not good for you either.

The bottom line here is that if you are ready and willing to go on a diet, then you have acknowledged the fact that you need to lose the weight and you are willing to do it. All that is left now is for you to be ABLE to do it and that requires you to IDENTIFY THE CAUSE of the weight – the psychological or mental factors that are causing you to eat the wrong kinds of foods and to eat too much of them – and then to go about dealing with those factors in a constructive way rather than the DESTRUCTIVE way (of overeating and eating the wrong kinds of foods.)

And there is NO SUBSTITUTE for exercise. Inactivity is the single most pervasive cause of obesity and general poor health in the United States today. Like it or not, you are going to have to get active somehow. Personally I hate exercise. I was a computer repair technician for years and then I taught certified computer repair technicians at the college level for many more years and all of these jobs, my career, involved working in air conditioned rooms on fixing computers, not stacking bags of concrete in some "unairconditioned" warehouse. I chose my profession because it was a nice indoor shirtsleeve environment. But once I decided to lose the weight I began taking the bus to work. This required a one mile hike to the bus stop and another one mile hike from the closest bus stop that I chose, to get to the campus. (There was a major bus stop on campus, but I chose to walk the additional mile from where I got off. There were indeed miserable times waiting for that bus in the heat and the rain, but I did it because I needed the exercise and I tried to walk briskly to get something out of it.)

But you don't need to hear my life story (it is admittedly rather uninteresting even to me) but you do need to get the exercise. If you don't want to go jogging or even walking down the street, then at least get some kind of exercise machine and do some sweating on it at least once a day. This is how we are built, we have to do some physical work or we simply wither away.

END OF CHAPTER QUIZ

1. The number one reason diets fail is:
    A. Diets are too hard to stay on them.
    B. Diets are too expensive.
    C. Diets treat everyone the same.
    D. They do not address the cause of your weight problem.
    Answer: D. The number one cause why most diets fail is because they do not address the cause of YOUR problem.
2. The physical cause of being overweight is:
    A. Eating the wrong kind of foods.
    B. Eating too much (excessive daily caloric intake)
    C. Lack of exercise.
    D. All of the above.
    Answer: D. All of the above. These three things are the physical cause of obesity.
3. The trouble with going on a calorie counting diet is:
    A. The 2000 calorie per day diet is a "one size fits all" number.
    B. The 2000 calorie diet does not take into account the form those calories take.
    C. A 2000 calorie diet could be a sudden and dramatic drop in the normal intake of calories for the dieter.
    D. All of the above.
    Answer: D. All three are contributing factors as to why calorie counting is generally an ineffective approach to dieting.
4. No matter how effective a diet might be, it will still likely fail because:
    A. People place unrealistic (too high) expectations on the diet.
    B. People consider it a chore and look forward to when it will end.
    C. There is no substitute for exercise which is necessary to lose weight and be healthy.
    D. All of the above.
    Answer: D. all of these are contributing factors to why most diets fail.

I am certainly not a psychologist, but I have been to them before and I can tell you that you will be a FAR HAPPIER person if you are ready and willing to face your closet full of skeletons. To acknowledge them is 90% of the battle towards defeating them. I have beaten severe hydrophobia by finally allowing myself to face the fact that I feared drowning because a neighborhood bully tried to drown me in a swimming pool when I was about 7 years old. Once I allowed myself to remember it and realized that this was just one event when I was a little kid, I got over it and learned how to swim and now I have no fear of the water at all (except for the deep ocean but that is my trauma from the original "Jaws" movie, a totally different problem!)

Some people need the professional help, I have needed it, and going to a psychologist right now in the 21st century really is the last of the unjustifiable bigotries of our society. As soon as you go to a psychologist and someone finds out, you are automatically stigmatized as some kind of lunatic and that is prejudice and bigotry of the most heinous and disgusting kind. But it is necessary in many situations because sometimes we have problems that are too difficult to bring up with friends and definitely too difficult to bring up with family (friends and family are usually the problem anyway!) Nowadays however, I don't care any more. I will bring up my problems with those closest too me because they either care enough to be helpful, and listening is usually all they need to do, or they don't care enough to help me in which case I decide that I no longer need them and they find themselves FIRED from my life.

I would rather have two or three good friends who really care than 500 "Friend me's" on bookface dot com or whatever the hell that crap is called. The point is that you are going to have to deal with your root psychological causes for the things that you do; especially to yourself. And if you think a session or two with a shrink will help – hey, I admit that I am as blunt as a brick up side the head – then DO IT.

In the mean time, I can help you in dealing with the physical causes of the weight problem. And the first thing we shall address is eating the wrong kind of foods.

DROP THE JUNK FOODS

In my own personal experience, I have over time dramatically reduced my daily caloric intake although I never actually counted calories, but I know the actual volume and quality of what I eat on any given day is far below what it used to be. And this is what we are addressing first: the QUALITY of the foods you eat. And this is the MOST IMPORTANT factor when it comes to weight loss and control not just for a few months but for the rest of your life and because you are going to drop the junk food and replace it with a

much healthier selection, the rest of your life will be a LOT
LONGER and HEALTHIER as well.

If you read the first chapter (STOP EATING POISONS) then
you know already part of the solution: do not eat those packaged
foods loaded with CANCER CAUSING CHEMICALS. There are
healthier choices even in potato chips (like baked ones rather than
fried) but they are all loaded with calories and you know you can't
be satisfied with having one "serving" of them (usually about three
– I jest but you know what I mean.) And there are those boxes of
individually packaged pastries and cakes, and boxes of cookies
and so on. And all of that junk is nothing more than addictive
mountains of junk calories that have no nutritional value and they
just keep piling up pounds and pounds of fat in your body and you
have to put a stop to that nonsense.

But, if you do throw all of that junk into the garbage can and
refuse to buy any more of it, then suddenly your body starts to
crave it – and that's when the trouble begins. So you can't just
stop snacking "cold turkey" either. Instead you must REPLACE
those awful mountains of JUNK FOOD, with mountains of
excellent HEALTHY snacking foods instead. Here are some of the
best choices:

1. **FRUITS** – You cannot go wrong if you replace those cookies
   and potato chips with fruits from the produce section of your
   grocery store. Fruits are nature's candy and the human species
   was literally raised on them. Ancient man's diet was about 90%
   vegetable or plant matter – mostly fruits – and about 10% animal
   matter. Fruits are loaded with vitamins and minerals and many
   other essential ingredients that our bodies need for proper
   health, I visit the produce section every time I go shopping and
   get whatever fruits are on sale at the time: bananas are
   particularly inexpensive, but just about everything the store
   carries goes on sale at some point and then I get them as well.
   But you can't buy too many because they can't sit around
   forever in the refrigerator. That brings us to the next choice.
2. **CANNED FRUIT** – As long as the cans are lined with plastic, so
   that the contents are not in contact with the metal, and most are
   these days, then this is an excellent alternative to fresh fruit and
   with the bonus that it does not take up space in the fridge. Only
   get canned fruit in "100% fruit juice" and not in "Light syrup" or
   worse "Heavy syrup." That garbage is corn syrup which is thick
   SUGAR and terrible for you. For that you might as well just buy
   the box of pastries and be done with it.
3. **FRESH RAW VEGETABLES** – Thin sliced carrot sticks and
   celery stalks are excellent snack foods. Do not be tempted to
   salt them or worse dip them in ranch dressing. I know how
   wonderful either garnish is for these, but the salt is terrible for
   your health (and messes with your heart) and the ranch
   dressing, even the low fat versions are thick because they are

full of oil (and raw egg which is TOXIC.) Oil is the room temperature liquid version of FAT. Yes, raw veggies are rabbit food and it takes some getting used to it, but over time I did and I am MUCH BETTER OFF and you will be too.

4. **SALAD** – A bowl full of raw spinach and lettuce with any other fresh veggies you might add like chopped onion, cucumber (skinned by the way, cucumber skins are not good for you either) bean sprouts (one of the very best foods for you by the way) raw snow pea pods (another food that is excellent for you) etc. is incredibly healthy for you. If you must garnish the salad, get some light olive oil, red wine vinegar and some spices (preferably fresh basil, oregano, cilantro, etc.) and make your own oil and vinegar dressing for your salad. Just read the labels (of the vinegar and olive oil and make sure they are NOT putting garbage chemicals into them.

5. **MAKE YOUR OWN** – For those who can really bake and make your own cookies and cakes from scratch: that is a problem. This is not what I mean. Because there are no such items in my house, then sometimes I make toast and eat it plain, but I mean 100% whole grain bread. And sometimes I do butter it, but the point is that it is still much healthier and it is far better than wiping out huge bags of potato chips and the requisite dip, or cookies and cakes and so on. It is better because I have to go through the effort of making it and nine times out of ten I will just make a salad or munch carrot sticks or crack open a can of peach slices instead. The point is that not having the junk food around forces me to find better things to eat.

6. **NUTS AND TRAIL MIXES** – Generally speaking, nuts are very good for you, but they are also very high in FAT and therefore calories. The far better choice is pumpkin seeds, sunflower seeds and pine nuts. I make my own trail mix predominantly out of shelled sunflower seed kernels, with some walnuts, almonds, and raisins added. For those who believe such a thing is expensive I get all of my ingredients at the local dollar store too and the resultant trail mix lasts me for many days even when I am hitting the batch a lot. I make up the whole batch and put it in a Tupperware and keep it in the fridge. All of the items in the mix are UNSALTED and the raisins must not be dusted with sugar either. The point is to drop GARBAGE food and eat HEALTHY food instead. We'll reduce the calories later.

7. **CHOCOLATE AND HONEY** – The first time I recommended this to a friend she thought I was insane. But I do not mean a chocolate candy bar: that is loaded with sugar, milk and a ton of other unhealthy nonsense. What I do mean is PURE 100% baker's chocolate or pure CACAO mass. You can find it in the baking section of the grocery store but READ THE LABEL. If it is loaded with junk like LECITHIN (animal FAT) it is garbage. You need to find the one with the ingredient label that reads "Cacao."

That's it; one ingredient. And in chocolate bar form. Now, it is BITTER. That's why I dip it in pure bee honey. So first let's examine the cacao. It has no calories from CARBOHYDRATES like starches or sugars and it actually has an unusually good effect on the human body – it is a natural antidote to many poisons. In fact it came into use a few centuries back by European royalty. They would eat it regularly because it would ward off the toxic effects of arsenic and other poisons which were being secreted into their food. Now for the honey: yes this is a complicated carbohydrate, essentially a very large and complex sugar molecule, so it does have calories, but it is also loaded with other extremely healthy substances: it has a natural and highly effective antifungal agent which is also perfectly edible and actually helps ward off fungal infestations in the human body. It also has a natural antibacterial agent which is also perfectly safe to consume and also helps ward off bacterial infections in the human body as well. The bottom line is that 100% cacao bars dipped in honey is one of the HEALTHIEST foods you could ever eat!

These are listed in order, the best choices are fresh fruits, vegetables and salads with your own oil and vinegar dressing followed by canned fruit, then nuts and dried fruits (like raisins) then an occasional indulgence of whole grain toast and finally the chocolate and honey. Honestly I can't find enough ways to eat pure bee honey. It is expensive I admit which is why I buy it the largest containers at the lowest cost per ounce that I can find. But it is so good for you, that you must incorporate it into your daily eating patterns. I also use it instead of syrup on my home made French toast: not exactly health food but I only make it once a week. Another thing I do is eat 100% pure peanut butter and honey either on whole wheat toast or straight off of the spoon – now that's a snack for a coach potato! Again, I do not wipe out whole jars of the peanut butter in one sitting, just a single piece of toast or a few spoonfuls at most; enough to get over the junk food craving until meal time.

The bottom line is that all of those cookies and crackers and snack cakes have been eliminated from my house, but whenever I crave them, I have an abundance of alternatives and seek out one of them instead. You can never go wrong munching on celery and carrot sticks and over time I have grown to like them and usually fall back to them unless I have a sweets craving, then I will hit the plums , grapes, bananas, raisins, grapefruits and so on.

REDUCING THE QUANTITY

This is the HARD one to deal with and that is exactly why I have loaded you up with so many healthy snack alternatives. It burns MORE calories to digest celery and lettuce, than they provide you. This is exactly why salads with only home made oil and vinegar dressing are my number one choice for snacking. The more celery you eat – the MORE WEIGHT YOU LOSE! Still it is necessary to get a handle on the snacking or overindulgence urges. And this cannot happen overnight. But over time I managed to pace myself and you can too. At first, just switch to the healthy snacking choices and restrict yourself to three meals a day and ONE snack in between. If that one snack for you consists of three apples, then so be it. Over time reduce that to two, then one.

The main objective here is that you are NOT ON A DIET; instead you are out to CHANGE your eating patterns for the remainder of your life from a very unhealthy eating regimen to a very healthy one. And that starts with changing the QUALITY of the foods you eat from very unhealthy choices to very healthy ones. Then having accomplished that, you can work on reducing your caloric intake, not by force, but by simply being aware of the concern and working to reduce the quantity of those foods that you know bring tons of calories with them like peanut butter and honey. I average one sliced banana in a bowl with one big dollop of peanut butter and a table spoon of honey about once every two weeks as a snack. Sometimes this is my breakfast and it is a lot healthier than a bowl of cereal which I haven't bought in years. Moderation in all things is the key to healthy eating habits; just don't try the cold turkey approach to reducing calories like my roommate. He ended up sucking down huge bags of popcorn and chips voraciously while convincing himself that he was on a "500 calorie per day" diet. That just can't be done and his body resisted the extremely low amount of food he was eating by skipping breakfast and having one little sandwich for lunch and one for dinner by giving him those cravings to shovel down all of those terrible snacks all day long in between the pitiful meals. And he convinced himself that those huge bags of chips only held a few hundred calories and conveniently ignored the "serving size" part of the nutrition label as part of the self-deception process.

EXERCISE

I hate exercise about as much as I would hate sleeping on a bed full of rattlesnakes. But there is no escaping the need for it either. One way or another you will have to break a sweat if you want to lose the weight.

The other part of this equation that I hate is having to do it in public. So I generally don't. On occasion I will walk the three mile round trip to my mail box (I live in a rural community and all of the mail boxes are in one place so the mail carrier doesn't have to drive a hundred miles of rock roads trying to find everyone.) Other than that I just jog in place until I break a sweat. And I do this several times a day. I am an old cuss with a long white beard like Gandalf in the movie "Lord of the Rings" so for me this is already plenty of activity. If you prefer to ride a bike or go swimming or even join a gym, that's fine too, but you have to do SOMETHING. And you have to break a sweat doing it: the harder you workout, the better. Now I know that a lot of people are quite overweight and don't want to be seen in public walking or jogging and I FEEL FOR YOU because I have been there. So you are going to have to bite the bullet and get some kind of exercise bicycle machine and you are going to have to get on that thing and use it and use it hard. The same roommate I have been telling you about got one of those "exercycles" and he did use it on occasion. It was a bit noisy, but I didn't mind at all. We all watched our TV on our computers with headphones which blocks out the sound anyway. If I couldn't keep up with my exercise regimen the way I am, I would definitely get one – no need for some huge high priced skiing treadmill contraption unless that's the one you want – and I would ride the thing for hours while watching my favorite programs.

As long as you recognize that there is no substitute for exercise and you realize that the only way any weight loss effort is going to actually work is if you exercise and if you begin to get active and find a way to do this, then and only then will you actually lose the weight and achieve your goals.

ON THE SUBJECT OF GOALS

Many people believe in setting goals and then striving to achieve them, and if that works for you then hallelujah. But every time I tried to lose weight and I went through this – weighing myself, setting the goal of my target weight, and then striving to achieve that goal – I would always become frustrated that this wasn't happening fast enough. In some cases I GAINED WEIGHT while trying to LOSE IT.

In the end, I stopped weighing myself and I stopped counting calories and I stopped trying to achieve very specific goals altogether. Instead I concentrated on improving the QUALITY of the foods in my daily eating regimen and then I started to REDUCE the QUANTITY of the foods I eat in my daily eating regimen and I put forth the effort to exercise and just concentrated on these things and IGNORED my weight and the number of calories I was eating and the GOALS and so on. All they do for me is create unrealistic expectations and that leads directly to FRUSTRATION which is soon followed by SURRENDER and FAILURE. But I did not want to surrender and I did not want to fail. And if you have made the hard choice to lose the weight then I am pretty sure that you do not want to surrender or to fail either.

Now if setting specific goals works for you, then go ahead and try it, but I will warn you that many people are go-getters who set goals for themselves and they work hard to achieve them and they are very accustomed to success in this way. Then they try the same method for success – setting specific goals – in dieting and they FAIL spectacularly. So what happened? How could such a dedicated person who did everything right and persevered with great sacrifice and hard work possibly fail? Answer: THEY made the decision and THEY made the sacrifice and THEY put forth the hard work and THEIR BODY simply refused to cooperate.

If it were so simple as to make the choice and do the work, then there would be no need for all of those diet companies selling all of their special milkshakes and pre-packaged meals and so on – a multibillion dollar a year industry in the United States. And if it were so simple then everything else concerning your own body would be equally simple too like getting over a cold, or even better, never catching one in the first place. But the fact is that our bodies are not subject to our force of will power anywhere near what we would like them to be. In philosophy there is something called the "mind-body problem" which incidentally has to do with metaphysics concerning what the Universe is made out of and has nothing to do with what we are talking about here except that it does have the perfect title for the dilemma we are facing as dieters: our body refuses to do what we want – it is NOT SUBJECT TO OUR WILL AT ALL. And in many cases, like mine, it will FIGHT YOU EVERY OUNCE OF THE WAY. It is the ultimate "Mind-Body Problem."

So rather than fight with my own body trying to force it to comply with some abstract number on the dial of some weight scale, I chose a different approach altogether: I will change the way I eat in particular, and the way I USE the calories I do eat, in a manner that is healthier and BETTER for my body. Then it will have NO CHOICE but to get healthier and to become more FIT as well. And as long as I ignore those numbers and those unrealistic expectations and stick to the plan: the part of the process over which I DO HAVE COMPLETE CONTROL – then sooner or later it is my body who will be forced to surrender – to give up those FAT reserves that it stubbornly hangs on to – and in the end I will win. And this ALWAYS WORKS because it is no longer a struggle and it is no longer a chore.

There are two ways to defeat an enemy: 1) Go to war and expend tremendous amounts of effort and tremendous amounts of time and resources or, 2) Make that enemy into your friend. So rather than spend all of the time, money and effort fighting with my body, I decided to make my body my friend. Instead of hating it and battling with it and trying to force it to comply with my wishes (my goals) I decided to be its friend and give it what it most desperately needs: QUALITY FOOD in the PROPER AMOUNTS and EXERCISE. And once I took up this mindset and totally forgot about worrying about my weight, it simply vanished as if it had never been there in the first place.

I first noticed it when a friend told me something like "Hey are you losing weight? It really looks good. Keep up what you are doing." And that was when it dawned on me that I had gone from using the first hole in my belt to the last one. And a few months later I had to buy new pants and a new belt to keep them up!

THE KEYS TO SUCCESS

NEVER GO ON A DIET. Instead set out to CHANGE your attitude from being at odds with your body – even hating it like I did – to understanding that the organism that your mind happens to inhabit is something different from your mind itself. An unhealthy body can certainly influence the mind in a negative way, and likewise the negative mind can certainly influence the body in a negative way, but the two are not as directly linked as we might believe or want.

But a healthy body can certainly lead to a healthy mind; and that would mean being happier and that can lead to peacefulness and contentment as well. And a healthy mind can lead to a healthier body too. But the body does have certain specific requirements and it does operate in a certain way. One of the most frustrating things about the way our bodies work is that it loves to be stuck in a rut. And when a person suddenly changes the quality and especially the quantity of food they eat on a daily basis, the body can and will fight back by hitting you with hunger and cravings and this can be a miserable thing to have to endure and this is why many diets fail.

Cravings often come from the fact that the body is used to a certain amount of calories and when it is denied those extra unnecessary calories it responds with hunger pangs even when the calories are not necessary, but the body loves that rut and tries to keep you in that rut. Cravings are also caused by the body when it realizes that it has run low on some essential nutrient, a vitamin, mineral or some other class of nutrient and it causes a craving for a specific food item that contains the nutrient the body needs.

It is amazing that such a thing is even possible. How does part of my brain know what foods contain some obscure substance like Omega-3 fatty acid, also knows that the body is low on it, and then causes in me a craving for fish? In other words, the body knows the things that are in our foods even when we haven't a clue. That means that there must be some kind of system at work, perhaps there are brain cells that actually detect the nutrients that enter the blood after each meal and they reference our cognitive centers, like language and vision and figure out what foods bring what nutrients. Either way, the process is obviously not well understood but it is also accepted by many in the medical field as a very real effect.

And we must train ourselves – our conscious selves – to recognize the difference between the body just trying to be a calorie hog stuck in that rut, and cravings that are based on the body's call for a specific essential nutrient because those essential nutrients cannot be ignored. In Volume 2 (The Truth About... Vitamins) I discuss the symptoms of the various Vitamin B deficiencies and they all sound very nasty – something to avoid. So a person might be suffering a craving for a nice big hamburger not just for the calories that the body has become accustomed to, but for the essential nutrients that it knows are in that hamburger and that it knows it needs.

And ALL diets are based on changing the foods that you eat on a regular daily basis. That means that all diets are going to change the levels of the nutrients present in your daily eating regimen. So even if the total calories of the diet were the same exact amount as before the diet began, their forms would be different (i.e. less carbohydrates and more protein) and the specific levels of the various essential nutrients will also be different. That means that if any one nutrient – even one science has yet to identify – is suddenly missing, your body will start to react by craving for it.

This is, in my opinion, one of the most prevalent causes of pervasive cravings and the misery of all diets. And it comes from the fact that science is in its infancy, we have only been doing science for about 400 years, but the human body has been around for tens possibly hundreds of thousands of years and the food we eat, like an apple, is so incredibly complex at the molecular level that we may NEVER KNOW the whole chemical inventory of a simple apple and we certainly will never know how all of those gigantic complex molecules function as a complete complex system of interacting molecules during our equally complex and unknowable digestive process.

We might some day be able to build a 3-D model of one of those gigantic molecules, just like we can make a model of a water molecule. But that lone H_2O molecule has a completely different behavior when you put trillions of them together. Together they form a water droplet which has a very different behavior from a single water molecule and the droplet has a very different behavior from an ocean of them. This behavior of complex systems is a field of mathematics sometimes called "Chaos Theory" because of the fact that so far we have had very little success in being able to predict the future behavior of any sufficiently complex system and the contents of our food, and the complexity of our digestive system, certainly qualifies as one of the most complex systems science is attempting to understand today.

This is the reason I always harp on eating raw fruits and vegetables the way they are found in nature; untreated, and uncooked. This is because mankind evolved eating them that way which means our digestive tracts are specifically built to get what we need from all of these foods in the exact form in which they are naturally found.

Likewise, any food that must be cooked, in order to make it edible, is something that we have only recently – since mankind's taming of fire – ADDED to our diet. This lowers their status from primary, necessary and desirable foods to secondary foods. This includes most beans, and roots like potatoes that must be cooked in order to be edible at all. Meat does not fall into this category because we cook it for another and even more important reason: to kill anything that might be in the meat like bacteria and even tapeworm eggs. So even though cooking the meat definitely changes it from the way it was found in nature for most of our evolutionary history, our ancestors discovered that by cooking it fewer of them got sick and died from eating it. So we must cook our meat and suffer the consequences of reduced nutritional value while enjoying the fact that it no longer kills us.

If we accept the fact that there are a lot of essential nutrients that we have yet to identify and any significant change to our food selection is going to cause this trouble, then we can at least try to prepare for this as best we can. An excellent method of preventing excessive difficulties like this during the change in food selection from BAD FOODS to GOOD ONES is to take supplements. If the body is receiving sufficient amounts of all of the vitamins and minerals that we know about, then we know that at the very least, any cravings that arise will not be caused by them, but by something else: either the basic craving for the additional calories which we are determined to resist until that goes away on its own – and it will – or some unknown nutrient present in those BAD foods which we have dropped.

The good news is that our digestive system is very resilient and resourceful. If some obscure nutrient is missing, we can make substitutions for many missing items and start using something else in our food that is available and synthesize what we need anyway. This process like everything else takes time and we may have to suffer through this process as well.

Our bodies use excess carbohydrates by storing them as fat. Basically our bodies are always trying to plan for lean times. This too is a result of all of those thousands of years as we evolved and ran into hard times often for days at a time with nothing to eat. So our bodies are very good at storing fat for a rainy day and they become very accustomed to doing this and as long as we never force our bodies to dip into those reserves, they will become very accustomed to that as well. And eventually our bodies will absolutely refuse to break into the emergency fat reserves and burn them up.

This however, is exactly what we want to happen when we go on a diet. But rather than just do it, the body reacts to a deficiency in caloric intake by hitting us with terrible hunger, demanding that we go out and get fresh new calories rather than break into the emergency reserves. It is incredibly frustrating whenever I reduce my caloric intake specifically to force my body to use up its fat reserves to endure the fact that it is so resistant to this.

Nevertheless, the only way to actually LOSE WEIGHT, is to BURN MORE CALORIES THAN YOU EAT. If that is not happening then you cannot and will not lose a single ounce. That is simple physics. Think of your fat as what I just described:

emergency fuel reserves that your body has carefully and meticulously set aside for hard times. And over a long period of time it has grown accustomed to setting aside the extra calories and it has also grown accustomed to never having to use them. So now you decide to start a diet and basically you are asking your body to break into those reserves and it absolutely refuses to do it. It will make you hungry and miserable and it will keep that up until you give in.

Eventually if you do hold out, your body will have no choice in the matter and it will break into those reserves and start to use them up. Once that process begins, you must force the issue and really make it burn off those calories. There are two approaches: 1) Sudden extreme reduction of caloric intake, and 2) A gradual decline of caloric intake. Both work, but you can guess that the sudden cold turkey approach will be difficult and miserable. I have tried both and they both work, you will have to decide for yourself which approach to take.

This brings up the exercise part of the equation. The reason this is necessary is because our muscles are the ones that do almost all of the major caloric consumption aside from the burning of calories to maintain our constant high body temperature. So if you do not change your daily routine to include some serious protracted activity, then your body has no reason to break into those carefully guarded reserves and burn up those stored calories. And bear in mind that whatever exercise you do, it has to last for a long time. Exercising for five minutes at a time will never work because your muscles have a small amount of stored fuel in them. Think of this as gasoline in the fuel line and the carburetor. When you turn the key to start your engine it fires up right away because there is gasoline in the carburetor and the fuel line – ready for immediate use. Our muscle cells also have fuel right there in them ready for immediate use too. This is called the "anaerobic" fuel supply. And this is what allows you to suddenly get up and go outside and check the mailbox and walk back into the house.

Your body continually replenishes the anaerobic fuel supply in your cells so that you can always MOVE. But it is short lived and once it gets used up then your muscles quickly and easily switch over to using the "aerobic" fuel supply. That is called blood sugar or glucose. And the muscles need to burn the glucose with oxygen, hence the term aerobic, this fuel needs air to burn it and so aerobic exercise is based on the fact that you workout long enough to exhaust your anaerobic fuel supply in your muscles and then you start burning the blood sugar. At that point you are going to have to start breathing heavier and it produces a lot more heat which is why you start to sweat. No long and protracted activity = no burning of aerobic fuel. Now you do not have an infinite supply of blood sugar either. So where will your body get the blood sugar from when it runs out? Answer: the liver.

The main job of the liver is to gather up all of the nutrients from your last meal and store them until needed then time release those nutrients into the blood and thus maintain its proper levels. As you burn up the glucose in your aerobic exercise, the liver releases more glucose into the blood and tries to maintain the proper blood sugar level. So what happens if the liver runs out of glucose? Now your body has absolutely no choice in the matter: it must start breaking up the stored fat molecules into smaller ones and those small units out of which those fat molecules are constructed are GLUCOSE molecules. So the ONLY WAY to coerce your body into giving up on those fat reserves is to literally force it to use them. And the ONLY WAY to do that is to engage in lengthy aerobic exercise. There is literally no other way. The good news is that you do not have to grunt and groan lifting monstrous weights on bar bells to make your body burn its fat reserves. But you do have to be active. If you are just going to walk, a very low energy activity, then you will have to walk for many miles before your liver runs out of its glucose molecules that it keeps on hand. So the more vigorous and energetic your aerobic workout is, the quicker you will burn through the anaerobic fuel in the muscles, the liver's glucose reserve on hand, and force your body to break into the fat molecules – the long-term fuel reserves – and start burning them up.

The diet product companies do not want to tell you that their products are essentially USELESS if you do not engage in serious aerobic exercise. If they did, then you would think "Why bother paying for your little pre-packaged meals when in the end the only way I am going to lose the weight is to exercise?" And you would be 100% correct. And that's why they extol the excellence of their products while conveniently ignoring this all-important truth.

If you have a very inactive lifestyle you should know that suddenly jumping onto a treadmill or an exercycle with the intent of working hard on it for hours could be disastrous. Your body is not accustomed to breaking into those fat reserves and will be very reluctant to do it at first, so reluctant that suddenly taking up a protracted and vigorous aerobics session could cause you to PASS OUT.

And those taking medication for blood sugar problems like hypoglycemia and diabetes are at very high risk for this. Like I said I am no doctor and if you know you have blood sugar issues (I have mild hypoglycemia myself although I have never taken medication for it) then do yourself a favor and consult with your doctor first. Just be plain about it and tell him you want to lose the weight and you want to do it with aerobics and let your doctor give you the proper course of action and give you any advice on safe guards that you can take in case you over do it.

My advice is to start by exercising up to the point that you begin to breath heavy and break a sweat and then stop. Time how long that took. Let's say it took five minutes. Now rest for one hour and repeat the exercise at the same intensity (this is why those devices like treadmills and exercycles are so handy) for the same five minutes. Do this three or four times a day, until it no longer forces you to break a sweat and breath heavy. Then increase the length of the activity until it causes the desired effect (break a sweat and breathe heavy.) Repeat that length of time three of four times a day until that is no longer enough to cause the effect and increase the length of the exercise session again and so on.

After several weeks of this, you have become accustomed to the extra work and your body will make many adjustments including preparation to tap into the fat reserves. Then you can try to reach the heavy breathing and break sweat stage and then push on for double the time. So if it now takes you ten minutes to start breathing heavy and break a sweat, continue at this level for another ten minutes with the understanding that if you start to feel WRONG in any way, then slowly back off and take a break for an hour and try again.

The whole point is that you must EASE INTO IT just like you should ease into the diet itself by first changing the kinds of foods you eat and then slowly back off the quantities of those foods.

THE KEYS TO SUCCESSFUL WEIGHT LOSS

1) **NEVER GO ON A DIET** – Instead CHANGE your eating habits for life by first improving the overall QUALITY of the foods you eat, and then by REDUCING the QUANTITY of the foods you eat. Be a friend to your body, not an enemy.

2) **AEROBIC EXERCISE** – IS THE MOST EFFECTIVE WAY TO BURN YOUR FAT RESERVES AWAY. Just like your eating regimen, you should ease into your exercise regimen as well.

3) **TAKE VITAMIN and MINERAL SUPPLEMENTS** - Hunger and cravings could be caused by the lack of an important essential nutrient when you suddenly start a new diet. To help reduce the potential for this take vitamin and mineral supplements starting on the day you make a radical change from the kinds of foods you used to eat to the new and healthier choices.

4) **WEATHER THE STORM** – Any time you make a significant change to the intake of environmental materials that your body depends on in order to survive, it will cause discomfort at the very least (death at the very worst!) Just think about breathing. Air contains oxygen which our body needs in order to live. Stop breathing and you will be dead in minutes. Since oxygen is all around us and abundant, this is why we have grown to be so dependent on it. But the food we eat is just as critical to our continued survival. Any person who stops eating will also die, just not as quickly, but it is just as guaranteed as if he had stopped breathing. So when you make a significant change to

what you eat and the amounts of it, it is logical to expect trouble so be willing to endure. Your body will get used to it and eventually like it.

END OF CHAPTER QUIZ:
1. All diets:
   A. Change the QUALITY of the foods you will eat.
   B. Change the QUANTITY of the foods you will eat.
   C. Don't address the need for exercise.
   D. All of the above.
   Answer: D. And this is the reason most of them fail.
2. All diets fail to take into account that:
   A. They don't taste as good as what you are used to eating.
   B. They are much more expensive than you can afford.
   C. The portions are too small to be effective.
   D. Sudden reduction in a nutrient could cause cravings.
   Answer: D. This is why I recommend taking vitamin and mineral supplements with any diet you try which ALL diet products fail to recommend.
3. No matter how effective a diet product might be, you will never lose any fat until you:
   A. Severely reduce your caloric intake.
   B. Change from eating bad foods to healthy foods.
   C. Get over the urge to eat too much.
   D. Exercise properly.
   Answer: D. While the rest might be true enough, you will never really force your body to burn those fat reserves until you force it to use them up. Exercise is the one way you can control.
4. The reason long vigorous aerobic exercise sessions are necessary is because:
   A. You have to get past the anaerobic and on-hand sugar supply in order to begin burning your fat reserves.
   B. It forces your body to burn a lot of calories and you must burn more calories per day than what you eat daily.
   C. Aerobics burns calories without actually body-building, so anyone can do it.
   D. All of the above.
   Answer: D. All of these answers are true.
5. You should immediately stop exercising if you feel:
   A. Pain or pressure in your chest.
   B. Light-headed or dizzy.
   C. Tingling in your extremities.
   D. All of the above.
   Answer: D. You MUST STOP EXERCISING IF YOU FEEL ANY UNUSUAL AND/OR UNCOMFORTABLE SYMPTOMS. IF THEY DO NOT GO AWAY PROMPTLY YOU SHOULD SEE A DOCTOR AND GET PROFESSIONAL ADVICE ON HOW TO PROCEED.

CHAPTER 4 – GOOD FOODS AND BAD FOODS

The first question on everyone's mind when I start to tell them that they do not have to buy into all of these diets and all they have to do is eat good foods and stay away from the bad ones is: "So what are the good foods and what are the bad ones?"

Obviously large bricks of pork lard are bad. But there are many bad foods that at first glance might not seem to be, and likewise there are plenty of good foods that people automatically assume are bad for you. Therefore it is necessary to spell out that bad list and then the good list with some explanations to help you make the right decisions. I have never liked to be told what to do and it got me into plenty of trouble as a kid, but once I was told WHY I was being told what to do and I was able to make my own determination that what I was being told was correct, then I happily agreed and complied every time.

THE BAD FOODS

1. **GRAINS** – Corn, wheat, barley, rice, etc. These have been touted as the large base of our food pyramid for the better part of a century, but this is a LIE. I already alluded to the problem in the previous chapter and now I will finish that argument. ANY FOOD THAT MUST BE COOKED in order to make it edible has been recently ADDED to our list of things we can eat and was not a part of our deep evolutionary history. So we spent millions of years evolving from whatever we were before, into what we are now and along the way, fresh uncooked plant products – fruits and raw vegetables – made up about 90% of our diet. Those foods literally raised us from monkeys to men and if they were good enough to do that, then they are still good enough to continue that process. In other words, our digestive tracts are made specifically to use those specific foods and so those are the primary choices. Anything that must be cooked was only discovered and added to our diet after we tamed fire, very recently in the grand time scale of our evolution, and thus these foods are only secondary at best. Corn is edible straight off of the stalk and that is my favorite way to eat it too. And cooking it does transform the hardened starchy kernels back into an edible form again, but these cereal grains should not comprise the majority of the foods we eat, but instead a minority of them. You can eat whole wheat bread, or even processed white rice, but only on occasion, and certainly not as the major bulk component of any meal.

2) **ROOTS** that must be cooked in order to be edible – Potatoes, yucca, malanga, boniato, etc. I know a lot of Hispanic folks will be upset by this one and Americans as well when it comes to potatoes. But the same problem exists for these foods as it does for the grains. If you have to cook it in order for it to become edible, then it was only recently added to the list of things we can eat and it was not a part of our deep evolutionary past. Again, you

can eat them, but not daily and not as the major bulk component of any meal.

3) **BEANS** and any other plant product that must be cooked in order to be edible – This includes chick peas, most kinds of beans that need to be soaked and boiled for hours, etc. It does not include green beans, and a few others that can be eaten raw (although they might not taste as good.) This is the same issue as the grains discussed above. I personally do not like the taste of raw green beans and I at least steam them a little but leave them crunchy. If you cook a vegetable for the taste, that is fine.

4) **BAKED GOODS** – Most are made with white flour unless explicitly stated otherwise and this stuff is basically as good for you as saw dust flour. While the bread makers have been much maligned for decades about their "white bread" products and have already been forced to offer whole wheat bread alternatives which are indeed much better for you, the fact remains that grains and their processed products like flour and all of the baked goods made from them are not good for you at all. But the fact remains that these products are bad for you for more reasons than just the grain flour out of which they are made. They also contain processed cane sugar or sucrose which is a disaccharide: it is two different sugar molecules bonded together: one glucose molecule and one fructose molecule. In your digestive system these are easily broken apart into the glucose and the fructose molecules. The glucose is ready to enter the bloodstream with no further chemistry needed, but the fructose molecules have to be converted into glucose which slows the process of absorption down. This is exactly why fruits are a far more healthy food even though they are very sweet; they contain fructose a much healthier version of sugar than sucrose. Baked goods also sometimes contain salt which we know is terrible: all salts cause the body to retain water and water retention can be a problem for many people. They also contain other salts (salts are a family of chemicals based on ionic bonding and there are many thousands of different salts) like baking powder or alum. Sodium aluminum carbonate contains aluminum which is suspected as being the cause of Alzheimer's disease. And our modern society puts this metal into every loaf of break and every can of soda pop. No wonder Alzheimer's disease is epidemic. Bottom line: try to reduce and better yet eliminate all baked goods that require white flour and alum – that stuff is potentially DEADLY.

5) **ANIMAL FAT** – Luckily cooking in animal fat and grease has been virtually eliminated in the United States and that is a very good thing. But ham hocks are still very popular in the South (where I am from, by the way) and this stuff is terrible. If our goal is to get rid of our excess body fat reserves, then eating animal fat straight up is the worst thing possible. Your body will carry those

molecules straight out to your thighs and store it – it's already in the storable form, so why mess with it?

6) **OTHER PROCESSED FOODS** coming from grains and inedible roots and their flours – Potato chips, potato bread, etc. They are worse than the plant products they are made out of, so don't mess with them.

7) **CANDY** – Nothing but chunks of processed cane sugar which is terrible for you. Eat fruit instead which is healthy for you.

8) **SODA POP** – This garbage is pure poison. You might not remember when you were a kid and had your first sip of cola, but I know what it did: it went right up into your nose and made you snort it out. The carbonic acid has no nutritional value nor do the carbon dioxide bubbles it produces to make the beverage bubbly. And another product with a red and white logo that shall remain unnamed includes phosphoric acid which will eat the rust off of a nail overnight. I don't know about you but I don't want that acid eating my intestines away. Then we have all of those artificial flavors, colors, sweeteners, etc. all of which are more likely to be CANCER CAUSING chemicals than not. Once in a great while I will have a root beer, but I have even eliminated that since there is nothing in it that was ever alive – they even stopped using the sapodilla tree roots to make it over half a century ago.

9) **SOY** – There is mounting evidence that soy beans and their by-products like soy milk are actually bad for you. I am not surprised by this since ALL BEANS are basically bad for you. If you are lactose intolerant or have switched to soy milk to escape from cow milk then try almond milk although unfortunately many people are allergic to almonds as well! Another interesting alternative would be coconut milk. It will certainly be sweeter than the other kinds of milk, but it is good for you. However, it does bring a lot of calories. Soybeans and their sundry by-products ranging from soy flour to soy lecithin, etc are showing up in almost all packaged and processed foods and they are potentially DEADLY. The food manufacturers use this TRASH because it is CHEAP GARBAGE FILLER. Refuse to eat any soy product and you will live a longer and healthier life.

RED MEAT, DAIRY PRODUCTS AND EGGS

Most people wonder why I haven't included dairy products or red meat or eggs in the bad foods list. The fact of the matter is that these are not evil foods, or I should say that they are not nearly as evil as the society would have you believe. I do agree that eggs are definitely a secondary type of food like potatoes because they must be cooked. Eating raw eggs, or specifically raw egg whites, is BAD FOR YOU. Something called "avidin" in the egg whites binds with many of those B Vitamins and prevents them from being absorbed in our digestive tract. It is so strong at binding to these vitamins that if another food you ate had them in it, it will bind up those molecules as well. Let's say that red meat, eggs and dairy products are all on the "EAT IN MODERATION" list.

GOOD FOODS

1) **EDIBLE RAW** vegetable LEAVES, STEMS, FLOWERS AND ROOTS – These are number one, the very best foods you could possibly eat and they should comprise the largest bulk component of your daily eating regimen. This includes lettuce, broccoli, cauliflower, carrots, onions, etc. Close relatives that are equally good for you are cabbage, bok choy, kale, leeks, asparagus, Brussels sprouts, celery, bean sprouts, alfalfa sprouts, spinach, turnip greens, scallions, snow pea pods, etc. I eat most of these raw but they are just as good for you steamed and still the best foods to eat even boiled.

2) **FRUITS** – Fruits are just as good for you as the raw edible veggies. These too are loaded with vitamins and minerals although the veggies do have a higher concentration of the minerals and other essential nutrients. Fruits are not limited to just those we think of quickly like apples, oranges, plums, bananas, grapes and watermelons. Watermelons are part of an enormous family of plants that provide us with many different fruits that we usually consider vegetables like yellow squash, zucchini, bell peppers and cucumbers. In fact, the whole family is sometimes referred to as the "cucurbits" and if you think about it for a moment, what does a watermelon look like? A huge cucumber! And while they are very distantly related and very different in taste, they are nonetheless related. Raw cucumber skin is not the best thing for you by the way. I usually thin slice off about half of it at least. Tomatoes are also fruits, though they are not related to the cucurbits, they are in fact a form of berry and I have a neighbor who grows a very small yellow variety that are as sweet as candy.

3) **NUTS** – Many nuts are loaded with vitamins and minerals that are rarely found in any other plant foods like vitamin E and some of the obscure minerals like magnesium and selenium can be found in some nuts. However, nuts are very high in calories due to their high oil content and they are definitely not diet foods. But they are still very healthy foods and should be included in moderation. Sunflower feeds, pumpkin seeds, and pine nuts are the better choices but still bring plenty of calories too. Peanuts are not true nuts but actually legumes like peas and they are at best secondary food sources because they really need to be cooked in order to be edible. The only thing I eat on rare occasion is 100% pure and natural peanut butter with honey. Coconut and white coconut milk as well as clear coconut water are also extremely healthy and good for you although unfortunately they too are not the dieter's best choice and bring a lot of calories with them.

4) **FISH** – This is the number one animal meat product. It is lowest in harmful fat and cholesterol and an excellent source of the protein our bodies need. Although most fish can be eaten raw I do

not recommend it. I had the unfortunate pleasure of having a marine biologist teach my Biology 1 class in college and his specialty was marine parasites. When we reached the phyla of the worms we got hour long slide shows of fish stuffed to the gills – literally – with worms of every conceivable size, color and shape. Cook your fish, trust me.

5) **POULTRY** (skinned) – the birds are also my number one choice for animal protein that our bodies need. Call fish number 1A and poultry number 1B. I know the chicken farms have been taking a lot of criticism and probably rightfully so for their treatment of the birds during their short and miserable lives in those places, and if you prefer to pay the extra for the "organic" chicken and turkey then so be it. I have replaced ground beef with ground turkey meat completely in my diet and properly spiced I have reached the point that it tastes to me every bit as meaty as ground beef and it is far better for you. There is some discussion about white meat being better than dark meat. While this might be true, I doubt that the dark meat (which comes from the legs of the chicken which do far more work in a **flightless** bird's life than the breast and wings) is actually bad for you. On the contrary, chicken, whether it is breast meat or thigh meat, is one of the very best forms of animal protein you can eat – just remove the skin which is heavy in fat.

6) **FRUIT and VEGETABLE JUICE** – Other than the occasional tea and my daily coffee (which I admit are NOT HEALTHY) fruit and vegetable juices should be your primary beverages throughout the day as well as water. Most Americans do not drink nearly enough plain and simple water and anyone on a diet should eliminate all other drinks except water. This will calm down the effects of osmosis caused by the excess of ionic compounds in your system (like salt) which causes water retention and bloating. As bizarre as it sounds, if you drink plenty of water, you will actually REDUCE that tendency. The only reason your body retains the water is because it must counteract the salts in your system and it feels that it is not getting enough on a regular basis. Once you do give your body more than enough water, it will relax its desperate tendency to grab as much water as it can when you do drink it. It also greatly helps your kidneys out and relieves the strain on them.

7) **YOGURT** – This is one of the healthiest foods you can eat. I highly recommend it as a healthy alternative to ice cream. There are many name brands and you should read the labels and make sure they are not sneaking chemical additives in there.

MORE ABOUT DAIRY

I have no quarrel with dairy products. They are edible raw and human babies are raised on milk whether it is human milk (the very best for them) or cow milk. It is difficult to know how far back our usage of animal milk goes but it is a fair bet that it really started when humans first settled regions and began farming and raising livestock. That is what we call the dawn of civilization about 13,000 to 15,000 years ago. Before that we probably never really got the chance to get milk from wild animals. This means that dairy products are likely a secondary food source at best. A special case of dairy products is cheese. This involves a special fungus that grows in the cream culture and gives it the particular texture, color and taste. Certain fungi, mainly mushrooms, are very good and healthy foods so there is no reason to believe that the ones in the cheese are any worse. I like cheese and I eat it on occasion, but beware, most kinds are not the dieter's friends and bring a lot of calories with them. The notable exception is cottage cheese.

ABOUT FRIED FOODS

The main trouble with fried foods historically was the need to fry them in animal fat. Now that we are using vegetable oil, that problem has been eliminated. The other trouble with fried foods is the breading. If it is based on white wheat flour then that is a serious problem. When I was growing up I never heard of gluten or anyone who couldn't eat bread or wheat flour products although I am sure those people were out there. Now I have heard about gluten and it seems that there are a lot of those people who cannot eat it. Gluten, by the way, is wheat protein and it is all that is left after they process the raw wheat and remove everything else of value and it is what we call white wheat flour.

It would seem that our population is resisting the fact that this stuff is in almost everything we eat from cradle to the grave and their bodies are literally screaming "That's enough already!" This is directly linked to the fact that about a hundred years ago Herr Haber, a German scientist, invented a cost effective way to get the nitrogen out of the air and into a usable form: ammonia. Nitrogen in the air is in the form N_2 which turns out to be an incredibly stubborn molecule that is very difficult to crack. But all life, especially plants need to get it and even they can't crack that nitrogen molecule. Luckily, the soil is full of nitrogen fixing bacteria who make their living cracking that molecule and releasing ammonia as a by-product of their chemical metabolism. The plants can then absorb the usable form and process it right into all of their molecules many of which are quite significant like the amino acids out of which all proteins are built. Even DNA is built out of amino acids.

Once Haber was able to manufacture huge quantities of ammonia, it was a simple task to manufacture ammonium nitrate – fertilizer. And once that happened farmers no longer had to let large tracts of their land sit idle for many years before they could plant again and the era of high intensity agriculture began and with it dramatically increased production of grains which directly led to the dramatic population explosion worldwide because our farmers were able to sell all of that grain to the rest of the world and we were now able to feed all of those people.

Now it turns out that this stuff is not the best food for humans at all. It's ok once in a while but not in every single meal, every day, all day, for generation after generation. Our bodies are quite literally getting FED UP with this excess of cattle feed in our diets and they are beginning to fight back.

I cook pork chops on occasion. That's certainly not a dieter's friend and not to be confused with health food either. But once a week or every other week I indulge myself. But now I skip the flour and just fry them straight up in the canola oil making them at least a tiny bit LESS BAD.

Another thing I love is fried okra. That's made with corn meal breading. Again, it's not to be confused with being good while on a diet, and certainly not the healthiest food on earth and that's why I only have it on rare occasion.

On the subject of canola oil, this is the ONLY cooking oil you should have in your house PERIOD. Canola oil is not just the healthiest vegetable oil for all purposes from frying to baking, it is actually so good for you that it would be worth drinking if it weren't so disgusting to do so. Canola oil by the way is derived from rapeseed. Someone at the company where they were planning to sell it decided that "Rapeseed Oil" would not have much market appeal and so they invented the beautiful name "Canola." Even rape plants are called Canola plants now! Rape is family to cabbage and grown for pig feed. It would be edible except for the fact that it turns out to be intolerably bitter (poor pigs.) But it is very fast and easy to grow for the pigs and the seeds are the source of one of the very healthiest vegetable oils on the market. Corn oil has calories and is a by-product of a grain which is a secondary food source at best. Olive oil is also very healthy but brings some calories and a strong taste which I only like on certain occasions. Peanut oil is very heavy and certainly not a diet food, but it does bring a wonderful flavor for frying foods.

The bottom line is that while on a diet you should definitely put away the frying pan until you have achieved the weight you want, and then only use it on rare occasions.

ABOUT PROCESSED MEAT

This includes hot dogs, Vienna sausages, bologna and so on. They all contain additives including nitrites in particular which are absolutely one of the worst chemicals you could ever eat. This is all basically junk meat, but if you can find lean versions with no nitrites in them (or any other chemical additives that are usually CANCER CAUSING agents,) then that would be ok on rare occasion. (I haven't found any nitrite free packaged meats yet.)

END OF CHAPTER QUIZ
1. Although loaded with vitamins and minerals, nuts are not the best thing to eat on a diet because:
   A. They contain toxins.

B. They contain salt which causes water retention.

C. They contain oils which are high in calories.

D. None of the above.

Answer: C. They contain oils which are high in calories. Nuts are very healthy for you, but only in moderation.

2. The very best beverage on Earth is:

A. Water

B. Fruit juice

C. Vegetable Juice.

D. All of the above

Answer: A. Water. They are all very good for you but water is the very best.

3. One of the worst beverages for you that most people think is good for you is:

A. Coconut water

B. Soy milk

C. Green tea

D. Almond milk

Answer: B. Soy milk. There is mounting evidence that soy beans and all of their by-products are bad for you. The rest are actually very good for you.

4. As far as we know, the following is not bad for you in moderation:

A. Beef

B. Eggs

C. Cheese

D. All of the above

Answer D. All of the above. These foods are not nearly as evil as they are portrayed and are excellent sources of protein, vitamins and minerals but only in moderation.

5. The reason fried foods are considered so bad is:

A. They were traditionally fried in animal fat.

B. The breading is made of secondary food sources and holds excess fat.

C. They all have too many saturated fat calories in them.

D. Both A and B.

Answer: D. Both A and B are the reason fried foods are generally considered bad for you.

6. Edible raw foods are the healthiest choices because:

A. They have least calories.

B. They are what our bodies evolved to digest.

C. They have more essential nutrients in them.

D. All of the above.

Answer: B. We are literally made to eat them.

CHAPTER 5 – THE PERFECT DIET

Before we begin I should tell you that I have three true diets for you to choose from and they ALL WORK and some BREAK one of my aforementioned rules: they make you count calories. Having said that, the difference is that I will tell you the TRUTH at every step of the way with no sugar-coating (that's bad for you anyway, right?) And I am not out to make a billion dollars by selling you diet products either.

EXERCISE IS A MUST

You must exercise and I do not mean walking so slowly that you never break a sweat or breathe heavily. You could walk a hundred miles on a cool autumn day and never breathe heavily or break a sweat. That means that you did all of that walking while only using the anaerobic fuels stored and continuously renewed in your muscle tissue. That means you are not forcing your muscles to run out of that fuel or the on-hand sugar reserves in your liver. And until you do force your body to run out of these reserves, you will never force your body to start burning its fat reserves and that is what MUST HAPPEN if you want to lose that fat. And if you don't force your body to tap into that reserve fat tissue then it will NEVER GO AWAY, PERIOD.

So you are going to have to start exercising BEFORE you start any diet whether you try one of mine or if you want to try someone else's diet, it doesn't matter. The only thing that does matter is that you MUST exercise PROPERLY and EFFECTIVELY or no diet on Earth will ever help you.

Now that we have that out of the way, let's begin.

EFFECTIVE WEIGHT LOSS EXERCISE PROGRAM

1. You must start exercising slowly. Ease into it. It doesn't matter HOW you exercise as long as one thing happens: during your workout you reach a point in which you start to sweat and breathe heavily. I don't like exercising in public so I jog in place in my home. But I do have weak ankles and sometimes I get a sprain (this has been a lifelong issue even when I was a skinny kid.) And if you are very overweight, you should definitely think about getting an exercise bicycle. Yes, they cost money but this is not a fad item that you will use for a few months and then throw in the closet to be forgotten; you will use it FOR LIFE. And it will bring you a much longer, happier and healthier life too. That makes it one of the best investments you could ever make. Just be sure it has adjustable resistance and try it out before you buy it. Once you reach that moment when you start to sweat and breathe heavily then stop. Take a break for about an hour and then repeat the process until you just break a sweat and start to breathe heavily. Do this three or four times a day with at least one hour in between.
2. Continue this process of exercising just to the point where you break a sweat and start to breathe heavily three or four times a

day until it takes you about 10 to 15 minutes to reach that point. Now once you reach that point, continue the exercise beyond that threshold for another 10 minutes monitoring yourself along the way. If you start to feel bad then certainly stop and take a break for at least an hour then try again.

3. If you can push through and exercise for an additional 10 to 15 minutes after you begin to sweat and breathe heavily do this three to four times a day. I know it is time consuming but I just bought some wireless earphones for my computer and I watch all of my evening TV while exercising: it is one of the greatest inventions ever. Persevere for about a week and now you are ready for the next step.

4. No more one hour breaks between exercise sessions. Now you will do one to two hours of sweating and breathing heavily continuously without a break or until you start to feel bad. If you do, go back to the previous method and continue that way until you wish to try again. Eventually you should be able to exercise vigorously for at least one hour straight and preferably two. You will get stronger and more capable of doing it as time goes on and in that case you can crank up the resistance if you have an adjustable machine so that you can get to the aerobic part (beginning to sweat and breathe heavily) faster and you don't have to spend as much time exercising but one hour is an absolute minimum and two hours is preferable.

At this point you are definitely forcing your body to tap into its fat reserves and now you are ready to begin your diet in earnest. Remember that you must persist with an exercise long past the point where you started to sweat and breathe heavily. With adjustable resistance exercise machines you can start with high resistance to get you to that point quickly and then back it off so that it still keeps you working hard but so that it doesn't kill you to keep it up for an hour and like I said repeatedly, two hours is better.

WARNING:

Another IMPORTANT REASON I urge you to ease into the exercise routine is because many people who are about to start losing weight have been overweight for a very long time. They have been eating bad kinds of food and too much food and been inactive for years possibly decades (like I was when I began) and that means that their cardiovascular health is also very poor. You don't want to buy a workout machine, jump on it and pedal it for two hours then collapse with a heart attack. Anyone regardless of their age who is significantly overweight and has been inactive for years to decades is at risk if they overdo it and I URGE YOU TO CONSULT WITH A DOCTOR BEFORE YOU BEGIN TO EXERCISE. Doctors can and will give you great advice on warning signs as well as explain to you how to monitor your heart with the devices they sell on the same store isle as the exercise machines, USE THOSE DEVICES AND BE CAREFUL.

TAKE SUPPLEMENTS

While exercising you should also begin to take nutrient supplements. I have gone out of my way to avoid using the word "multivitamins" for a reason: almost every product I have checked has many unusable or unacceptable ingredients in it – even the big name brands. Any of these "A to Z" products are certainly better than taking nothing at all, but they are definitely NOT the best choices. "The Truth About… Vol. 2 – Vitamins" will direct you on how to find the best vitamins and you should take all of them. . "The Truth About… Vol. 3 – Minerals and the Other Essential Nutrients" covers those and you should take all of those as well.

The reason for this as already explained is that when you make a radical change to the KINDS of food you will be eating, you change the quantities of these nutrients and your body has gotten accustomed to the levels in your old eating regimen. And when they change, your body will immediately fight back with cravings and that is the primary TORTURE of dieting. By providing your body with ample amounts of all of these essential nutrients you are basically eliminating this problem before it even begins.

This means that most likely the cravings you will be suffering once the diet begins in earnest will be due to your body craving the extra calories that it is also accustomed to and those are the cravings worth SUFFERING THROUGH in order to reach the optimal levels of caloric intake. In other words, because our bodies love to be stuck in a rut, or they become ADDICTED to anything and everything we do, they also become ADDICTED to excess calories and the only way to get over any ADDICTION is to SUFFER THROUGH THE WITHDRAWAL.

Taking vitamin, mineral and essential nutrient supplements helps curb these cravings and personally I am surprised that no one (that I know about) has ever mentioned this.

DIET #1 – "WEANING OFF THE BAD STUFF"

By the time you start any diet your should already be exercising properly (see the section above) and taking a good regimen of daily vitamins, minerals and essential nutrients. At this point, it is time to start whatever diet you want to try and it will be HIGHLY EFFECTIVE.

This is a simple diet and works as follows:
1. If you are a heavy junk food snacker, this is target #1. And it must END. See the previous chapter on healthy snacks to replace the junk food but to quickly recap: 1) Carrots and celery (no garnish of any kind – no salt, no dip, just plain,) 2) Any other raw edible vegetables (usually a salad with a SMALL amount of oil and vinegar dressing ONLY.) 3) Fruits (sparingly because they do have a LOT of sugar in them which we really DO NOT WANT,) 4) Low calorie snack foods like YOGURT. And of course the complete

elimination of junk food stuff like snack cakes, cookies, potato chips and so on.

2. Pick ONE MEAL and change it into the HEALTH meal of the day. If it is breakfast then whatever it was before, change it to a few fruits – especially a grapefruit (fully ripe with NO SUGAR ON TOP) a banana (by the way, they do not have enough potassium to satisfy your daily requirement) and one other item like an apple. For the drink, coffee is a very bad habit to beat (I never have) so use milk or creamer sparingly and sweeten it with a touch of honey (at least it is far better for you than cane sugar and not a DEADLY CANCER CAUSING CHEMICAL like all of those terrible artificial sweeteners. If you can pass on the coffee then drink green tea if you need or want a hot beverage and low sodium tomato juice is the very best. The low sodium version of these products uses POTASSIUM salt instead of sodium salt to get its salty flavor. YOU NEED THAT POTASSIUM and it does contain MORE of the adult Recommended Daily Allowance of potassium (FAR MORE than bananas.) One grapefruit whole, one banana or two, and one apple accompanied by a 12 oz. bottle or carton of low sodium tomato/vegetable juice is the perfect breakfast.

3. After a week or two change the second meal in the day to a healthy one: For lunch a tossed green salad with a touch of oil and vinegar dressing is IDEAL.

4. After a week or two change the third and final meal of the day to a healthy one: You might have noticed that you haven't had any meat all day. Now you can indulge because you DO NEED ANIMAL PROTEIN in your diet contrary to the beliefs of the fanatical vegan fringe. Only one or two individual and very specific plant food sources contain sufficient levels of two animal amino acid in them, otherwise plants are very LOW on them. Not to mention the B vitamins and many other complex molecules that we have yet to even identify or understand their roles in our bodies. If you are a fanatical fringe vegan then God bless you I am not telling you that you are wrong, just make sure that you are getting those nutrients that is deficient in most plant matter. See the section above on the run through of the good foods but the very best would be baked or boiled fish, or skinless chicken with a side of steamed vegetables (that are edible raw like broccoli, green beans, etc.)

At this point you MUST NOT BE CONCERNED about the PORTIONS of these very healthy choices that you are eating at each meal. If you are sticking strictly to carrots and celery as your snack food – which I did when I started – then you have gone a LONG WAY to reducing your daily caloric intake often by as much as 5000 less calories per day!

Drink mostly water throughout the day rather than soda pop, and add in a little green tea or fruit juice to break up the monotony. This for many people also eliminates thousands of calories. If you drink artificially sweetened soda pop, at least it is not bringing calories with it so you could continue to do that, but I HIGHLY RECOMMEND that you drop that CANCER COCKTAIL and start drinking water first and fruit juice and low sodium vegetable juice as the second choices.

NOW REDUCE THE PORTIONS

The finishing touch on Diet #1 is to begin to reduce the portions of those things within your diet that bring the most calories, that would be the fruits and the animal products, Replace them with raw edible vegetables instead. Don't completely eliminate them, just cut back. 4 to 8 ounces of meat per day is all that a healthy adult human really needs.

DIET #2

This one is exactly the same as the one above in that you must change junk food snacking into health food low calorie snacking and change each meal one at a time into a healthy low calorie alternative. In this version the only difference is that for each meal you can replace it with any of the myriad pre-packaged diet products on the market like those complete frozen dinners. This is a much easier diet to pursue since the meal is already prepared and ready in a few minutes in the microwave oven and the calories are printed right on the package. If you replace your breakfast with a diet packaged meal that says it is 600 calories that is excellent. Eat the salad for lunch when you change that meal out to better food. And eat the prepackaged dinner product. If that is also 600 to 800 calories again that is perfect. In this way, you can be sure that your caloric intake is KNOWN and far lower than it was before you began.

DIET #3 "ALL OUT WAR"

WARNING: THIS DIET IS DANGEROUS. SO PROCEED WITH CAUTION.

It works because I have done it and I lost 60 pounds in 40 days and that is no exaggeration. In fact, I used to live in a high rise condo on Miami Beach and another resident got into the elevator with me one day and said, "Excuse me, I don't mean to intrude, but I am a medical doctor and I have noticed that you have lost a LOT of weight over the past few weeks and just wanted to ask you if you are alright."

If you do this, it will work alright, but it makes you lose weight TOO FAST; so fast in fact, that you must be careful. And you must drink nothing but water while you are on it, and you must drink VERY LARGE QUANTITIES OF WATER while you are on it. Any time you shed weight like this you are forcing your body to use up fat reserves that have been built up over many years and they are loaded with additional stored things in them like excess CALCIUM. Once freed and not used, it will go to the kidneys to be removed and too much CALCIUM can give you KIDNEY STONES and from what I have heard from people who have had them – they are not exactly fun. YOU HAVE BEEN WARNED.

The diet is very simple: eat nothing but whole grapefruit and celery. That's it. You are allowed three grapefruits per day, peel and eat them like an orange and never put sugar on them. If you must put an artificial sweetener on them, to be able to tolerate them, then go ahead and do it. You can eat as much celery as you want and you will be CRAVING and HUNGRY ALL DAY so you must also take a complete regimen of vitamins, minerals and essential nutrients as well and you must drink nothing but water and LOTS of it.

Ironically, exercise is not even required for this diet to work although I highly recommend that you undertake the exercise regimen that I described at the beginning of this chapter and be well into it before you try this diet and also be prepared to lighten up on your routine because you will actually be CONSUMING A NET NEGATIVE TOTAL CALORIES PER DAY. This is in fact exactly how this diet works and why it is so effective and powerful and DANGEROUS.

Remember I mentioned that it takes MORE CALORIES to digest celery than what it gives you. So if each celery stalk takes 200 calories to digest and yields 100 calories to your body to use, then the more of it you eat, the more calories you LOSE doing that. The three grapefruits are an ESSENTIAL part of this diet. Grapefruits contain a very specific enzyme only found in them that actually PROMOTES THE BURNING OF FAT in your body. So while they do provide some sugar, it is not enough to keep you from having to dip into your fat reserves. AND it helps and promotes the burning of those fat reserves – this diet is like firing both barrels of a double barrel shotgun at the same time. So even if you spent decades sitting around eating tons of junk food and barely moving like I did back then, the diet will literally carve the fat right off of your bones.

THE FINAL ROUND OF WARNINGS FOR DIET #3:

If you are over 50 years old YOU SHOULD NOT TRY THIS DIET. TRY #1 or #2 instead. You will note in those diets that I am recommending a whole grapefruit for breakfast – the food that has the enzyme that promotes and encourages your body to break up its fat reserves, and to snack on celery all day because it provides you with a NET NEGATIVE caloric intake. Every celery stalk you eat equals calories LOST not gained. You could call Diet #1, my Diet #3 "Lite."

If you are taking ANY MEDICATION including but NOT LIMITED TO: high blood pressure medications, cholesterol, hypoglycemia, diabetes, or heart medications THEN DO NOT ATTEMPT DIET #3 AT ALL. Anyone on those medications MUST CONSULT WITH THEIR DOCTOR BEFORE STARTING ANY WEIGHT LOSS

PROGRAM THAT INCLUDES STRENOUS EXERCISE AND A
CHANGE IN THEIR DAILY FOOD REGIMEN.

END OF CHAPTER QUIZ

1. The MOST IMPORTANT thing to do on a diet that does NOT
involve food is:
    A. Take vitamin, mineral and essential nutrient supplements.
    B. Exercise properly.
    C. Drink plenty of water.
    D. All of the above.
    Answer: D. All of the above are NECESSARY in order to make
        any diet EFFECTIVE.
2. The #1 source of excess calories in many people's daily eating
habit is:
    A. Excessive snacking on junk foods
    B. Eating too much of the wrong kinds of foods at meals.
    C. Bad choices in beverages (i.e. soda pop, coffee with cream
        and sugar, etc.)
    D. All of the above.
    Answer: A. Excessive snacking on junk foods, although the
        others are just as bad and many people are overweight
        because of them too.
3. The two best foods to eat while on a diet are:
    A. Apples and bananas.
    B. Fish and skinless poultry.
    C. Grapefruit and celery.
    D. None of the above.
    Answer: C. Grapefruit and celery. The others are good for you
    and good for dieters, but grapefruit has the enzyme that
    promotes the breakdown of fatty tissues in the body and
    therefore encourages the body to break into its fat reserves and
    use them up. Celery provides a NET NEGATIVE number of
    calories, so every celery stalk you eat is like eating –100
    calories; the more you eat, the more weight it causes you to
    LOSE.
4. Losing weight too fast is DANGEROUS because:
    A. Fat tissues not only store fat, but also other nutrients
    including calcium that can cause kidney stones in excess.
    B. Rapid weight reduction can put a strain on the cardiovascular
    system.
    C. Rapid weight loss can result in dehydration.
    D. None of the above.
    Answer: A. Large amounts of fat being dissolved for use as fuel
    also releases other essential nutrients stored in those tissues
    including calcium. Too much calcium in the blood can cause
    kidney stones.

The most important thing to remember is that dieting is about losing weight. And just like making money, or any other endeavor that you might pursue; there are highly effective ways to do it and there are highly ineffective ways to do it. Putting a million dollars into a Certificate of Deposit at the bank will make money, but only a small trickle of it. Using it to build a fast food franchise will make TONS of constant and guaranteed cash flow. Likewise, you could keep cutting back on the amount of food you eat and you could improve the quality of the food you eat daily, and this will certainly help, but it is NOT HOW TO LOSE WEIGHT. For that you MUST burn away your fat reserves and that requires long vigorous AEROBIC EXERCISE sessions. That is the most effective way we lose weight and you can control how many calories you burn each day. As long as it exceeds your daily caloric intake then you will be, by definition and in keeping with the laws of physics, losing weight.

It is important to know how our bodies work and what they were made for (if I add this extra phase it will prevent the sentence from ending in a preposition like I am supposed to.) We were made to toil. There is no way around that. But in our modern high tech society, many of the good paying jobs require us to work in an air conditioned office sitting at a computer all day long. This does not mean that those jobs are easy, just different – no toil. But toiling all day is what our bodies are made to do and if denied this, they atrophy. One of the principle methods in which our bodies decay over long periods of disuse is that they gain weight in the form of accumulated fat, they lose muscle mass and tone, and the cardiovascular system decays including a weakening of the heart and a build up of plaque on the arterial walls. Inactivity KILLS. And heart disease is the #1 cause of hospital visits and DEATH in the United States today and one of the primary causes of it is INACTIVITY – lack of proper exercise.

The other causes include: poor diet, chronic lack of sufficient vitamins, minerals and essential nutrients (don't forget that we are the best fed, and most MALNOURISHED society the planet has ever seen) and poisons like alcohol and cigarettes.

The #1 reason most people decide to go on a diet is to improve their appearance which is a dreadful mistake. I cannot imagine personally going through all of that hard work and suffering to satisfy the needs of a world of perfect strangers who do not care if I am alive or dead. Certainly for me being obese got a lot of attention, negative and unwanted attention to say the least. But when I got rid of it I found that I got no attention at all. Once I was lean, people then found me unremarkable and totally ignored me. That is the very BEST a person can hope for if they do the hard work and the suffering of losing weight: they will get ignored.

Now, that is blissful compared to the stares and the snickering behind my back I assure you, but it is still not enough to justify all of the time, sweat, money, pain and suffering of enduring a diet. That is why you mustn't "go on a diet" at all, but instead CHANGE your daily eating regimen from a bad one to a healthy one, and couple that with proper exercise so that your new and improved eating patterns will help you lose the weight.

And the REASON to change one's lifestyle and make those sacrifices and do that hard work and endure all of that suffering should never be for a population of strangers (to hell with all of them, they never mean to help you; only to criticize and hurt you.) Instead, change your eating habits and start exercising for YOURSELF. Weighing upwards of 70 to 80 pounds less than I did FEELS wonderful. I am old and decrepit now, and a lot of the time I suffer back pain and knee and ankle trouble from a life time of injuring them while toiling at hard jobs all of my life, but I cannot imagine the misery I would be in right now if I had to put all of that extra weight on those joints today. I doubt seriously that I could even get out of bed.

But the reason it feels better is precisely because you will BE BETTER. Not just lighter, but also HEALTHIER. It makes you stronger, nimbler, gives you far greater endurance, greater resistance to disease and chronic illnesses like heart disease, diabetes, and so on. And this superior health and fitness makes you happier as well and the greatest gain of all is that you will live longer. Now it is not desirable, as far as I am concerned, to live longer if it is going to mean ten extra years of total misery. The good news is that having lost all of that weight and maintaining a better, healthier eating habit and exercise regimen, I feel better physically as well as emotionally than ever before, so those extra ten years or whatever extra time I get by living healthier is spent in RELIEF FROM PHYSICAL MISERY, and in HAPPINESS.

You know what it is like to be sick with a cold or flu. It is miserable because you are physically UNWELL. And all you can think about is getting over that cold so that the physical suffering will end. I am not about to say that being obese is a disease, but it is a state of being physically UNWELL. Not just because you have to lug around all of that extra weight, but also because of the fact that the human body was not meant to be obese and the causes of it: poor diet, poor nutrition and inactivity are what are making you obese which is to say: UNWELL. And losing the weight in the ways described in the preceding chapters will change your life primarily because you will go from a state of being UNWELL to a state of being WELL. Basically you will go from being physically AFFLICTED by a chronic MALADY, to being RELIEVED of that AFFLICTION or you can call it a RETURN TO GOOD HEALTH. And that IS worth all of the hard work and suffering it takes to make that happen I assure you.

I harp quite a bit about two things: exercise and eating raw edible foods. The exercise is because the human body was made to toil as already expounded upon quite enough, but the raw edible fruits and vegetables are also just as important. Just as we were made to toil, we were also made to eat these exact foods. Our evolutionary history (and trust me I am not a big fan of the "theory" of evolution, but that is a subject for another book!) goes back a very long way and before man discovered and controlled fire and then discovered how to use it to cook, all we ever ate for all of those tens to hundreds of thousands of years was raw edible food. Our digestive tracts are made exactly for those foods and not anything else.

We cook food, which chemically transforms normally inedible foods like potatoes and rice, into foods that we can digest, but they are still not a part of our deep evolutionary history, so our bodies do find a way to use the transformed chemistry from cooking them into usable nutrients but they are definitely not the first and best choices and we do suffer if we rely too heavily on these kinds of foods which have only been ADDED to our available food source list recently – within the last 15,000 to 35,000 years at most. Plenty of time it would seem for generation after generation to "evolve" the capacity to consider them primary food sources but apparently that has not happened. Because in the last 100 years our science and technology took a huge leap forward with the Haber process allowing us to manufacture fertilizer for the first time in our history which allowed us to produce huge excesses of food for the first time in our history.

So in the last hundred years these secondary food sources that need to be cooked in order to become edible like wheat (and dairy products because we can now raise many more heads of cattle than ever before) have become our primary food sources and the population is SUFFERING BADLY because of it. Lactose and gluten intolerance are showing an ever-increasing rise to the point of reaching epidemic proportions because our digestive systems are not made for these foods and more and more people's bodies are starting to fight back and reject them completely.

I understand that many people do not particularly like the raw edible vegetables. And my own personal favorite and sizable side dishes throughout my whole life were potatoes slathered in butter and rice with gravy: two TERRIBLE secondary foods bathed in TERRIBLE secondary food garnishes adding up to huge amounts of UNHEALTHY FOOD SOURCE calories. So I want you to know that I suffered HORRIBLY making the transition of food choices in my own life from those wonderful tasty foods to what amounts to rabbit food. It is interesting to note that rabbits have almost the exact same nutritional requirements as humans and can only eat what we can eat. So calling my meals "rabbit food" is not an insult, it is simply scientifically correct. There is no doubt about it, dropping all of those grains and inedible raw roots is hard work, but over time I have grown to like my new healthier choices and you can too. Although honestly, I have never really grown to like celery, but if I must snack, then it is the best choice for health reasons and because I don't really like it that much, I don't eat very much of it either. It just helps me get over the snacking urge until meal time.

Celery should probably be called a spice. And there is a whole huge shelf of spices at the grocery store and many of these spices (other than salt of course and a few others) are pure plant products most of which are edible in their fresh raw form. I would personally never sit down to eat a bowl of fresh green basil – the flavor is a bit too strong for that! But I do add it to my oil and vinegar dressing along with many other spices. Many of these have essential nutrients and curative substances in them as well. Learning to use them in my cooking has gone a long way toward helping me to tolerate my new food choices. Being Italian seems to have given me a genetic love for Italian food which seems absurd but I sure do love it. And I have restricted myself to eating pasta only once a month because of the wheat flour in those noodles. But my love for garlic has helped me eat all of the other food choices as well. The bottom line is that if you do not like the taste of some food then CHANGE IT: SPICE IT UP. My friends can no longer be in my kitchen because of the heavy miasma of spice fumes in the air while I am cooking and they can't even get near a plate of my food any more, so I do admit that my taste buds have been ruined by this tendency, but you certainly do not have to go overboard with spices like I have in order to spice up your foods and make them at least "less bland."

I have no quarrel with vegetarians or the radical militant vegan extremists: to each his own as they say. The only criticism that I have is that almost all plant matter is short on 2 essential amino acids – methionine and lysine which must be in the foods we eat (that's why they are called essential nutrients.) The point is that our bodies either can't make them, or don't make enough and they are in plant foods in reduced quantities is why vegetarians don't shrivel up and die, but think about this: if a contractor has to build 100 houses but only has the bricks to build 50, and is therefore forced to make wooden molds and pour the concrete into them to make the bricks for the other 50 houses it will take a lot more work and take a lot longer to get the 100 houses built. It is a well known fact that a high protein diet facilitates healing of injuries. This is because new cells must form and grow at the injury site and if they have all of the building blocks on hand, then they too can get that work done faster and easier than if they had to make those building blocks from scratch.

But that is certainly not the extent of the problem. Almost all of our organs, from the skin to the bones as well as the liver, kidneys, etc. all continuously renew themselves. It is estimated that over a period of 27 months your liver is made of almost all new cells. Obviously it is an ongoing process, so this is an average over time. The only organ that does not do this is the brain. If it kept changing out old cells for new ones then how could you remember things you did in your childhood, memories that are permanently stored in specific brain cells? Because of this constant renewal of almost all of our tissues, providing the cells with ALL of their building blocks greatly facilitates this effort and that is why a small daily portion of animal products is recommended even if it is technically unnecessary. It just removes an additional step of work that those tissues would have to perform in their absence.

And vegetarians and vegans may not be 100% correct in their dietary habits if they are eating tons of grains which are only SECONDARY food sources and should be in the "few and far between" minority of the foods we eat; not the vast majority of the bulk of our daily food intake.

I have no quarrel with pork meat either. But again it should be classified as the fourth choice behind fish, then skinless poultry, then beef, then pork. Processed pork meat such as hotdogs, sausages, etc. is out of the question. They contain nitrites and other terrible deadly chemicals and are mostly fat. That is the worst thing to eat regardless of whether you are on a diet or not. Thin sliced pink ham in moderation (that means about 4 to 8 ounces per meal (depending on your size) once a week or two is fine. But not in a WHEAT BREAD sandwich. Now you are combining TWO secondary food choices making the whole meal BAD. Instead I slice it up and add it on top of a salad along with a few sliced hard boiled eggs and a sprinkle of sharp cheddar cheese and turn the whole thing into a Caesar's salad which serves as both a late lunch and an early dinner all in one. It's not about the foods themselves, it is about the portions when it comes to proper healthy eating habits.

While fish is certainly number one, there are very healthy fish and very heavy oily fish. The good news is that even the heavy types of fish like mackerel, sardines, and tuna are still FAR BETTER choices than any other kind of meat. All of that fatty oil is the good kind, low on saturated fat (beef and pork fat are nothing but saturated fat which is terrible for you and chicken fat is right up there too) and it is high in polyunsaturated fat which is the GOOD KIND of fat and it is loaded with excellent additional essential nutrients for your body like the Omega-3 fatty acids which promote heart health and are ESSENTIAL nutrients too.

If all you ever ate from now on was fish you would be certainly on the right road to eating a very healthy diet.

I would be remiss if I did not talk about these forms of fat and the other dirty word that has come to prominence since the 1980's: cholesterol.

Fats and oils are related at the molecular level; they are very similar. If the molecules are large enough and also have very few double bonds between the carbons in those massive molecules, then this is what we call a saturated fat and it will be a waxy solid at room temperature. This is the animal fat found in beef, pork and chicken and it is what is in our fat tissues as well. It is a very compact high energy food source, but unless you are very active, then all of that saturated fat will be quickly transported out to your thighs and stored rather than get burned up and that is why you should greatly reduce the amount of it in your diet. Technically it is not bad for you, it just brings far more calories than most people would ever use and excess calories get stored making animal fat a very fattening kind of food.

Polyunsaturated fat, on the other hand means that there are many double bonds between the carbon atoms in the fat molecules. These tend to be thick liquids at room temperature which we call oils. These store a lot lower amount of energy for one, and they can also be broken down and serve as basic building blocks for other molecules that the cells need to manufacture, so far less of these polyunsaturated fat molecules end up being stored as fat in our bodies and serve as low level construction material for our tissues instead: that's why these are the GOOD KIND of fat.

SECTION OF A SATURATED FAT MOLECULE:

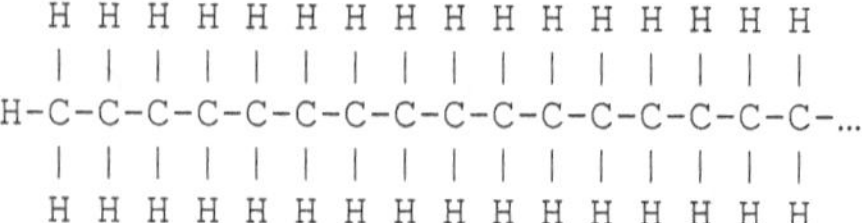

In this molecule each Carbon atom along the chain is bonded with a single bond to each neighbor leaving two free bonds for hydrogen atoms to occupy.

SECTION OF A POLYUNSATURATED FAT MOLECULE:

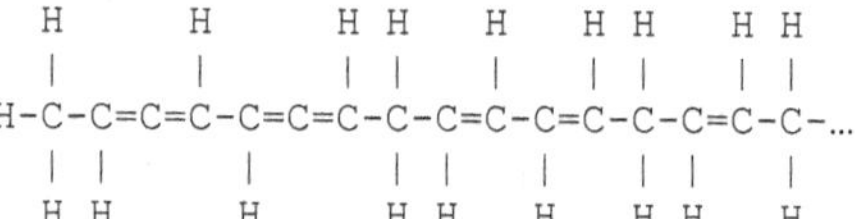

In this molecule there are double bonds between some of the carbon atoms in the chain, since each carbon atom only has four bonds, each double bond costs bonding locations for hydrogen atoms, so there are far fewer of them in the molecule. This is where the saturated fat molecule gets its name: the carbon chains are saturated with as many hydrogen atoms as they can possibly hold. Polyunsaturated fat molecules mean that there are many double bonded carbons so there are many "holes" where hydrogen atoms are missing from the molecule.

These are enormous molecules that can contain hundreds of carbon atoms and other elements as well (mostly oxygen which is why they are called carbohydrates) and the structures can be branched too. The point is that saturated fats hold a lot of potential energy for burning. In fact the same molecule but with only eight carbons in a simple chain is what chemists call octane, the most flammable component of automobile gasoline and a gallon of it can move your car upwards of 20 miles at tremendous speeds. So a small amount indeed holds a lot of stored potential energy. But the saturated fat molecules are much more massive than the polyunsaturated ones and tend to slip and slide past each other less readily than the less massive polyunsaturated ones. This is exactly why saturated fat like the white marbling in beef and pork as well as chicken fat blobs are solid at room temperature while the polyunsaturated fats are liquids – oils – at room temperature and also why if you heat animal fat it melts readily. The weight difference between the two types of fat molecules is just barely enough to keep saturated fat solid at room temperature.

I bring all of this up to point out that for decades food manufacturers have been turning the good polyunsaturated fat molecules into the BAD saturated ones. They take a vegetable oil – a polyunsaturated fat that is GOOD FOR YOU – and "partially hydrogenate" it. The chemical process removes some of the double bonds in the polyunsaturated fat and adds more hydrogen. This makes the oil heavier and therefore it becomes a solid at room temperature. They have invented artificial ANIMAL FAT THAT IS BAD FOR YOU and they are putting it into a lot of different foods.

My objections to this garbage are myriad and sundry. You know I don't trust ANY CHEMICAL dreamed up and cooked up by mankind in a chemistry lab in my food because that was invented within the last 60 years but our bodies have been around for tens to hundreds of thousands of years and they are built to digest what we have been eating all of that time – NOT THE GARBAGE we just started cooking up in those test tubes. Chances are if we cooked up the chemical it is a DEADLY CARCINOGEN. Second, they just turned a HEALTHY FORM OF FAT – the polyunsaturated fat – into a BAD FORM OF FAT – a saturated fat called a "trans fat" since it is an artificial hybrid molecule that MAKES YOU FAT and causes your LIVER SERIOUS PROBLEMS.

Any product label that contains any ingredient that reads "Partially hydrogenated" (or "hydrolyzed" is another way to say the same thing and try to hide what they are doing,) then DO NOT BUY IT AND DO NOT EAT IT. All of these companies have only ONE OBJECTIVE: to make money. As consumers, the more people who stop buying their CANCER COCKTAIL GARBAGE, the more they will be inclined to stop putting it into our foods. We have already seen this in the fact that these companies now offer us 100% whole wheat grain bread, and line those infernal tin cans with an inert plastic so the contents don't taste like the can and give us metal poisoning.

The more we say "No" to Yellow #5, sorbitol, BHT, and the list goes on for miles, the more they will realize that we don't want to eat that DEADLY CANCER CAUSING GARBAGE any more.

Where to begin with the cholesterol fiasco? About 30 years ago researchers learned that high levels of cholesterol – another form of fat by the way – were directly linked with heart disease and heart attacks. They immediately got the word out that eating this stuff was DEADLY and the one food with one of the highest concentrations of it is eggs. And so the campaign began to convince everyone that eating eggs would kill you. Oh, and by the way, beef and pork are also laced with it so stop eating those as well.

My knee-jerk reaction to this was to go out to a restaurant and order a nice steak and eggs breakfast. I did this because these jokers are the same ones that never make a peep about the endless studies that show Yellow #5 is a CONFIRMED CARCINOGEN. So they seem to believe that eating Yellow #5 is safe and eating natural food is DEADLY? In my personal opinion that makes them ignorant or evil and I don't bother listening to either kind of person… I stopped taking advice from idiots and demons long ago. Think about it, they are essentially saying that manna came from hell and whiskey comes from heaven. Now, I might be a Southern redneck, but I am not THAT stupid, come on!

And it tuned out that I was right. After a few years they discovered that there are TWO kinds of cholesterol: High Density Lipids (saturated lipids and lipid is a fancy word for "fat") or HDL's and Low Density Lipids (unsaturated form) or LDL's. And the LDL's are the ones that are bad for you and the HDL's are GOOD FOR YOU (opposite to the kinds of regular fats, by the way.)

Now, there is no denying the fact that the primary culprits that get blamed for people having high cholesterol (beef, pork, and eggs) are loaded with BOTH and should be cut down and even avoided for a time if a person has high BAD cholesterol levels, but one of the BIGGEST problems with cholesterol is that people do not know what it is FOR or where it comes from (ends in a preposition I know. Shouldn't verbs that require them like "Comes from" be exempt?) So what is cholesterol for? It is the lubricant between all of your individual muscle cells that allows them to lie in a bundle and slide easily past each other as they contract and relax causing us to move. And WE MANUFACTURE IT OURSELVES FOR THIS PURPOSE. So if you never consume even one single molecule of cholesterol, your body (your liver makes it by the way) will still be loaded with it so that you can move. And you could still have high cholesterol including the bad LDL levels in your blood.

Although I must admit that if a person ate nothing but steak and eggs for breakfast like I did for years, then they would have a much higher tendency to have high cholesterol (like I did) and by eliminating these foods, they have a very high likelihood of eliminating that problem, but the fact of the matter is that a person could still maintain this high cholesterol level once their body gets accustomed to it. And that is a problem.

But there are ways to correct this. And most people do not know how, and this is the reason that some people might be suffering from high levels of the bad cholesterol: Vitamin B3, a.k.a. Niacin. Niacin BLOCKS the PRODUCTION OF THE BAD FORM OF CHOLESTEROL. And it is an ANIMAL VITAMIN rarely found in plants and even when it is there, it is usually in trace amounts that would force you to eat a truck load of the plant in order to get enough of it. Ironically, beef and eggs (properly cooked with no runny egg whites) are the best natural sources of Vitamin B3! Anyone suffering from high cholesterol – and this is purely a personal opinion – should get off of the cholesterol medication and start taking Vitamin B3 instead. This is FAR BETTER FOR YOU since most of those dangerous medications' manufacturers are now being SUED due to harmful side effects (like DEATH of the patient as a result of taking that garbage) and in a few years all of the new ones will be the topic of lawyers' commercials all day and night as well. Just take Niacin supplements (indeed take a whole Vitamin B Complex to make sure you get all of these ESSENTIAL VITAMINS) and be done with it – and of course eat the healthier foods I have outlined in this book and EXERCISE.

THE BOTTOM LINE

Each day a person consumes a certain amount of calories and they burn a certain amount of calories. If that person consumes MORE calories than they burn during that day, then they will GAIN WEIGHT. Our bodies are fanatical about storing calories, any excess calorie will get stored, not thrown out; our bodies are simply too efficient to do something like that. So you only have TWO choices on how to CHANGE this arrangement: 1) You can REDUCE your caloric intake until it goes below what you burn each day, 2) You can INCREASE the number of calories you burn each day so that it surpasses the amount you consume.

For inactive people, reducing their caloric intake until it is below what they consume is, in effect, a starvation diet similar to DIET #3. The only difference with DIET #3 is that it does allow you to eat all the celery you want, but it will still be MISERABLE (the person will be constantly hungry and wracked with cravings for "real" food.)

The second method is FAR BETTER for you and FAR MORE EFFECTIVE: to take up exercise and increase the number of calories you burn each day so that it surpasses the number of calories that you consume.

Each diet in this book is a COMBINATION of the two: REDUCE your daily caloric intake AND increase the number of calories you burn each day. And this is GUARANTEED to work: its physics. If your car gets 20 miles to the gallon and has 5 gallons in the fuel tank and you drive it 100 miles you will run out of gas and the car will come to a halt. Likewise if you burn more calories than you eat each day then your body will have NO CHOICE but to break into your fat reserves and start to burn them up. And thus you WILL LOSE WEIGHT.

FINAL WARNINGS AND DISCLAIMERS:

1. While I don't have a PhD in medicine or anything related to it, I have researched everything that I purport in this series over the course of the last 35 years (since I CHANGED my own lifestyle.) I just can't remember which page of which book I read in 1985 that had the specific fact that I am now spouting. But I did go through the trouble at some point to look it up and VERIFY the source FIRST before I started applying the information to my own life.

2. I did all of this research for me and never thought about the fact that someday I would write a book about it so that's why I never kept any notes either. The bottom line is this: YOU DO NOT HAVE TO TAKE MY WORD FOR ANYTHING I SAY: I WELCOME AND ENCOURAGE YOU TO LOOK THESE THINGS UP FOR YOURSELF.

3. What I do have is 35 years of experience in eating healthy and researching foods, both good and bad, and what they have in them (that is good or bad,) and the nutrients and the diets and in applying them to my life. So I have a LOT OF PRACTICAL EXPERIENCE about what works, what doesn't and WHY that is.

4. USE ALL INFORMATION PROVIDED IN THIS BOOK AT YOUR OWN RISK. But I say that so no one will come out of the woodwork and try to sue me because they killed themselves trying Diet #3 AFTER I REPEATEDLY TOLD EVERYONE THAT IT IS DANGEROUS.

END OF CHAPTER QUIZ

1. ALL diets usually FAIL because:
   A. They only address half of the cause of a person's weight problem (their daily food intake.)
   B. They fail to mention that lengthy vigorous aerobic exercise is the most effective method of losing weight and returning to optimum health.
   C. They fail to mention that a good daily regimen of vitamin and mineral supplements can greatly reduce hunger and cravings while restricting a person's daily caloric intake.
   D. All of the above.
   Answer D. These are the three main reasons why almost all diets fail to work.

2. Which of the following should be considered "secondary foods" and severely limited from ones daily food regimen?
   A. Potatoes
   B. Rice
   C. Most kinds of beans.
   D. All of the above.
   Answer D. Anything that must be cooked in order to become edible is a secondary food added to our potential food sources after the dawn of civilization and we did not evolve to eat these foods.

3 By far, the best possible animal meat is:
   A. Pork
   B. Eggs.
   C. Ground turkey.
   D. Fish.
   Answer: D. Fish is by far the best possible source of animal meat.

4 Unsaturated fats:
   A. Have more double bonds in the carbon chains.
   B. Fewer hydrogen atoms in the molecule.
   C. Are the healthy form of fat.
   D. All of the above.
   Answer: D. Unsaturated fats have extra bonds between the carbon atoms and therefore fewer hydrogen atoms in the molecules and these are the GOOD forms of fat that we can use in our bodies.

5 The best way to reduce the bad form of cholesterol in our bodies is to:
   A. Reduce it in our diet (less beef, pork and eggs)
   B. Take niacin supplements
   C. Stay active and exercise regularly.
   D. All of the above.
   Answer: D. Stick to this plan and you can avoid having high cholesterol for life.

6 The ONLY way to lose weight is:
   A. Reduce the number of calories you eat each day
   B. Increase the number of calories you burn each day
   C. Burn more calories than you consume each day.
   D. Eliminate sugar and saturated fat from your diet.
   Answer: C. Burn more calories than you consume each day. A, B, and D, will certainly contribute to this effort.

THANK YOU AND GOD BLESS AND GOOD LUCK AND ABOVE ALL ELSE: TAKE CARE OF YOURSELF (BECAUSE NO ONE ELSE IS GOING TO DO IT)!